EPIDEMIC

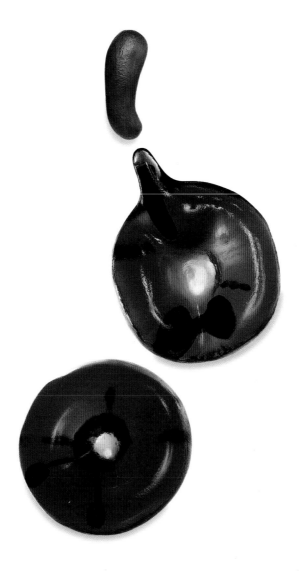

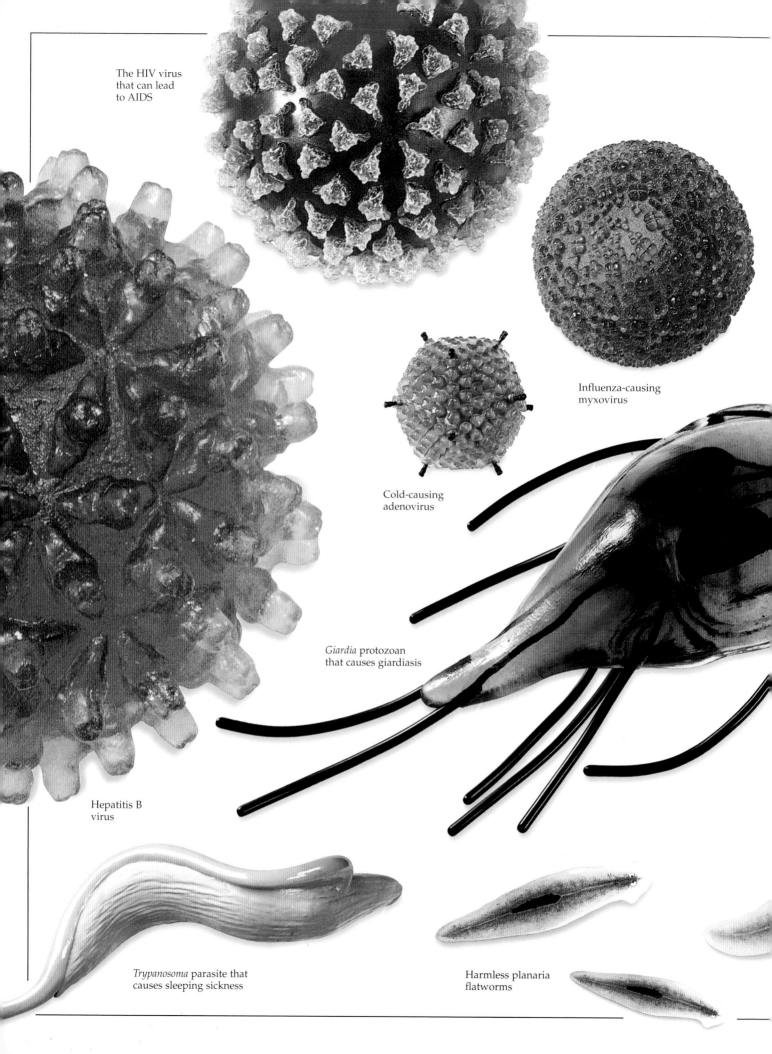

The HIV virus that can lead to AIDS

Influenza-causing myxovirus

Cold-causing adenovirus

Giardia protozoan that causes giardiasis

Hepatitis B virus

Trypanosoma parasite that causes sleeping sickness

Harmless planaria flatworms

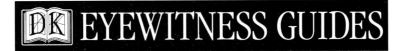

EYEWITNESS GUIDES

EPIDEMIC

Written by
BRIAN WARD

Chief Editorial Consultant
DR ROB DeSALLE
Curator, American Museum of Natural History

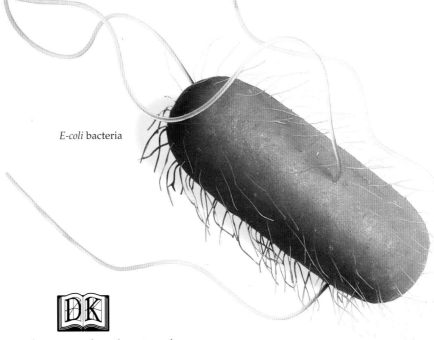

E-coli bacteria

A Dorling Kindersley Book

IN ASSOCIATION WITH THE
AMERICAN MUSEUM OF NATURAL HISTORY

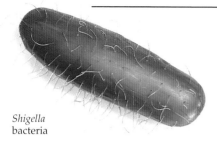

Shigella
bacteria

Light
microscope

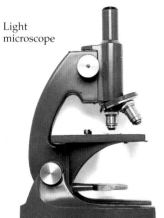

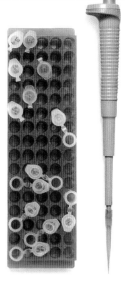

Immunity testing equipment

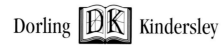

Dorling **DK** Kindersley

LONDON, NEW YORK, SYDNEY, DELHI, PARIS,
MUNICH, and JOHANNESBURG

Project editors Ann Kay and Carey Scott
Project art editor Joanne Connor
Managing editor Sue Grabham
Senior managing art editor Julia Harris
Production Kate Oliver
Picture research Samantha Nunn
Senior DTP designer Andrew O'Brien
Jacket designer Margherita Gianni
Special photography Denis Finnin, Jackie Beckett, and
Craig Chesek from the American Museum of Natural History

This Eyewitness ® Guide has been conceived by
Dorling Kindersley Limited and Editions Gallimard

First published in Great Britain in 2000
by Dorling Kindersley Limited,
9 Henrietta Street,
Covent Garden, London WC2E 8PS

2 4 6 8 10 9 7 5 3

Copyright © 2000 Dorling Kindersley Limited

A CIP catalogue record for this book is
available from the British Library.

ISBN 0 7513 2871 5

Colour reproduction by Colourscan, Singapore
Printed in China by Toppan Printing Co., (Shenzhen) Ltd.

See our complete
catalogue at
www.dk.com

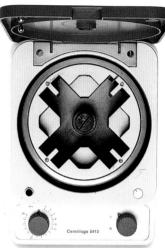

Sterilization unit
for disease
research
equipment

Sample tubes

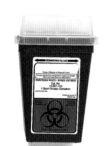

Disposal unit for
bio-hazardous
waste

Streptococcus
bacteria

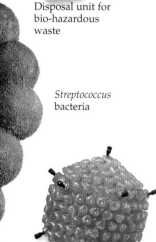

Adenovirus

Laboratory
equipment

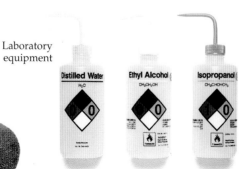

Bilharzia
flatworm

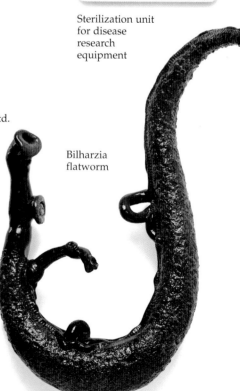

Contents

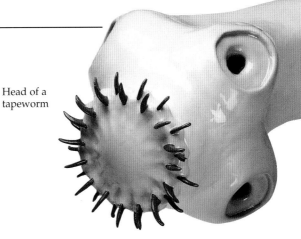

Head of a
tapeworm

What is an epidemic?

INFECTIOUS DISEASE HAS ALWAYS existed, around both humans and animals. Ever since people began living in communities, disease could pass easily from one person to another. Often, only a few people become ill. When, however, the problem spreads outside a limited group, affecting a large number of people and lasting for some time, it is called an epidemic. If it becomes established right across the world, then it is a pandemic. Diseases that are present all of the time are said to be endemic – for example, malaria is endemic in certain tropical regions. Infectious disease is caused by micro-organisms such as viruses invading the body. Also known as microbes, these micro-organisms are carried in various ways, such as via animals or through the air.

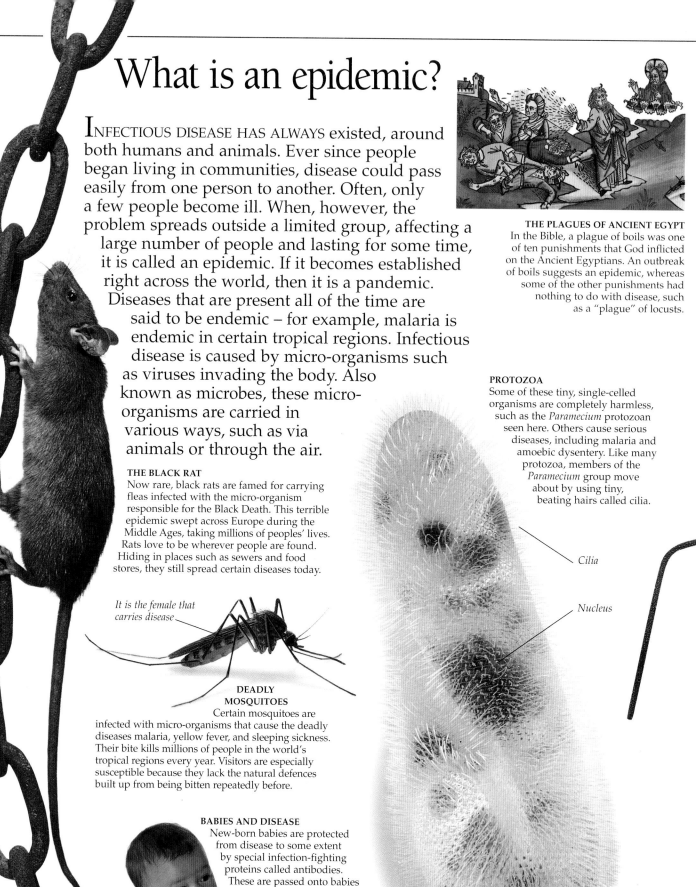

THE PLAGUES OF ANCIENT EGYPT
In the Bible, a plague of boils was one of ten punishments that God inflicted on the Ancient Egyptians. An outbreak of boils suggests an epidemic, whereas some of the other punishments had nothing to do with disease, such as a "plague" of locusts.

PROTOZOA
Some of these tiny, single-celled organisms are completely harmless, such as the *Paramecium* protozoan seen here. Others cause serious diseases, including malaria and amoebic dysentery. Like many protozoa, members of the *Paramecium* group move about by using tiny, beating hairs called cilia.

Cilia

Nucleus

THE BLACK RAT
Now rare, black rats are famed for carrying fleas infected with the micro-organism responsible for the Black Death. This terrible epidemic swept across Europe during the Middle Ages, taking millions of peoples' lives. Rats love to be wherever people are found. Hiding in places such as sewers and food stores, they still spread certain diseases today.

It is the female that carries disease

DEADLY MOSQUITOES
Certain mosquitoes are infected with micro-organisms that cause the deadly diseases malaria, yellow fever, and sleeping sickness. Their bite kills millions of people in the world's tropical regions every year. Visitors are especially susceptible because they lack the natural defences built up from being bitten repeatedly before.

BABIES AND DISEASE
New-born babies are protected from disease to some extent by special infection-fighting proteins called antibodies. These are passed onto babies from their mothers. This protection wears off, however, and while young children develop their own antibodies they are very vulnerable to infection.

Paramecium protozoan

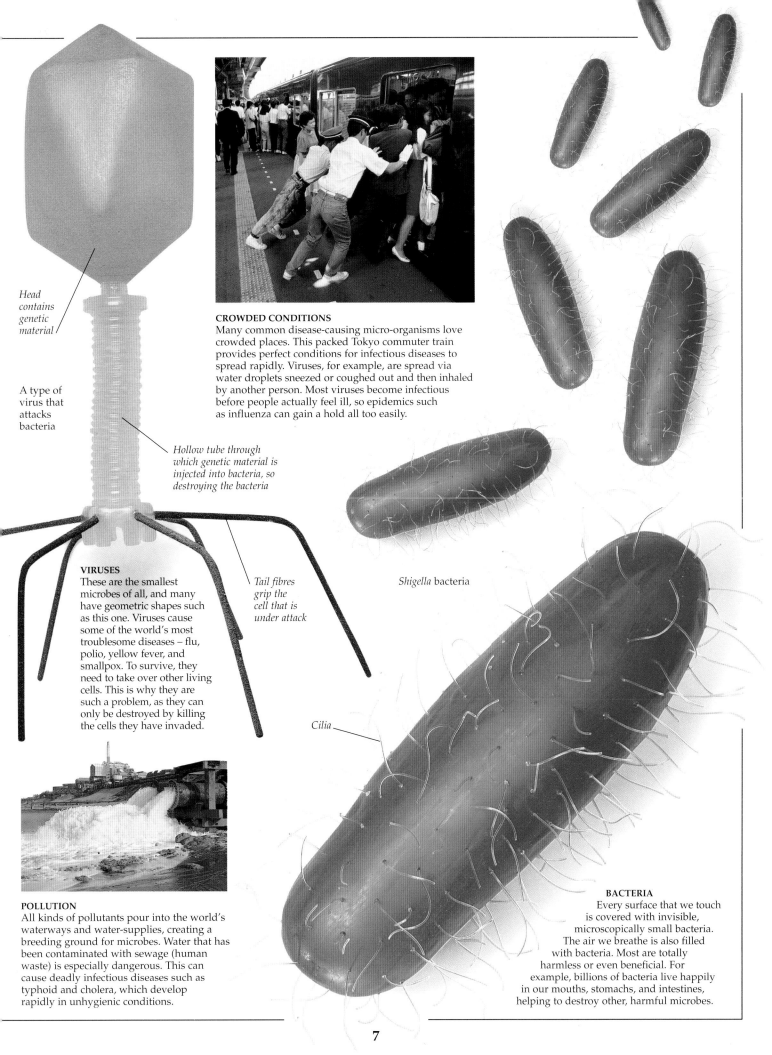

Head contains genetic material

A type of virus that attacks bacteria

Hollow tube through which genetic material is injected into bacteria, so destroying the bacteria

Tail fibres grip the cell that is under attack

CROWDED CONDITIONS
Many common disease-causing micro-organisms love crowded places. This packed Tokyo commuter train provides perfect conditions for infectious diseases to spread rapidly. Viruses, for example, are spread via water droplets sneezed or coughed out and then inhaled by another person. Most viruses become infectious before people actually feel ill, so epidemics such as influenza can gain a hold all too easily.

VIRUSES
These are the smallest microbes of all, and many have geometric shapes such as this one. Viruses cause some of the world's most troublesome diseases – flu, polio, yellow fever, and smallpox. To survive, they need to take over other living cells. This is why they are such a problem, as they can only be destroyed by killing the cells they have invaded.

Shigella bacteria

Cilia

POLLUTION
All kinds of pollutants pour into the world's waterways and water-supplies, creating a breeding ground for microbes. Water that has been contaminated with sewage (human waste) is especially dangerous. This can cause deadly infectious diseases such as typhoid and cholera, which develop rapidly in unhygienic conditions.

BACTERIA
Every surface that we touch is covered with invisible, microscopically small bacteria. The air we breathe is also filled with bacteria. Most are totally harmless or even beneficial. For example, billions of bacteria live happily in our mouths, stomachs, and intestines, helping to destroy other, harmful microbes.

How an epidemic evolves

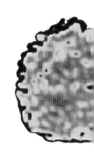

WHY IS IT THAT EPIDEMICS appear, then gradually die out? This process has been going on for thousands of years, with new diseases causing widespread illness and then seeming to disappear. One reason for this is that the microbes that cause disease are constantly changing. Another important reason becomes clear when diseases that previously lived only in animals suddenly spread to humans. Our immune systems have no resistance to these new diseases. If the outbreak occurs in a crowded city, sickness spreads rapidly and the infection quickly develops into an epidemic. As an increasing number of people become exposed to the disease, the immune system learns to fight off the infection. As more people become immune, the disease becomes less of a threat.

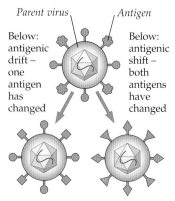

ANIMAL CARRIER
The monkeys that carry yellow fever, and the mosquitoes that feed on them, naturally live high up in the forest canopy. However, as the human population has increased, forests have been cleared. Infected monkeys have come closer to humans and infected mosquitoes have spread the disease by biting people.

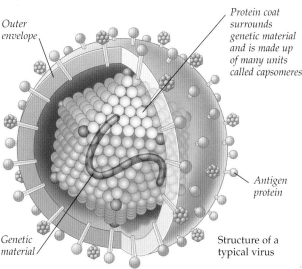

Outer envelope

Protein coat surrounds genetic material and is made up of many units called capsomeres

Antigen protein

Genetic material

Structure of a typical virus

INSIDE A VIRUS
A virus consists of a strand of genetic matter enclosed by a protein shell. The genetic material allows the virus to copy itself once it has invaded a living cell. Some viruses also have a protective outer layer. The virus's surface is covered with proteins called antigens. These lock on to a host cell, enabling it to be invaded.

Parent virus *Antigen*

Below: antigenic drift – one antigen has changed

Below: antigenic shift – both antigens have changed

HOW VIRUSES CHANGE
When a virus reproduces it can alter its antigens. The body's immune system recognizes a virus by the antigens on its surface. If these change, the virus may go undetected. A small antigenic change is called an antigenic drift. A larger change is called an antigenic shift and may lead to an epidemic.

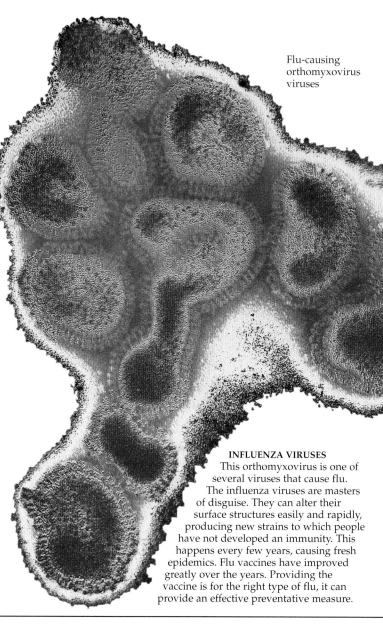

Flu-causing orthomyxovirus viruses

INFLUENZA VIRUSES
This orthomyxovirus is one of several viruses that cause flu. The influenza viruses are masters of disguise. They can alter their surface structures easily and rapidly, producing new strains to which people have not developed an immunity. This happens every few years, causing fresh epidemics. Flu vaccines have improved greatly over the years. Providing the vaccine is for the right type of flu, it can provide an effective preventative measure.

Several yellow fever viruses, which belong to the flavivirus group of viruses

YELLOW FEVER VIRUS
This virus was once found only in animals. Yellow fever in humans was first described in 1684. The spread among humans was started by travellers and explorers who had been bitten by mosquito carriers while abroad and then took the disease back to their homeland. Yellow fever is often mild, but it may be fatal. Symptoms include fever and jaundice, which makes the skin turn yellow – hence the name. One attack gives immunity for life. The yellow fever vaccine has been highly successful in controlling this disease.

FOREST DANGER
Felling forests is just one of the factors that can cause disease. When trees are cut down, microbes and parasites can easily move from forest animals to humans. Disease-causing organisms usually live in their original hosts without too much harm. However, if they come into contact with people who have no immunity to them, they can go on to cause disease. The ways in which environmental changes can affect the course of disease is a vast area of current research.

Cubic shape, despite looking rounded here

RICE-PADDY BREEDING GROUNDS
Water-filled rice paddies provide ideal conditions for mosquitoes to breed. Mosquitoes can carry yellow fever, malaria, and dengue fever, which they pass on when they bite people working in the fields. Rice is a staple food for half the world's people. As the human population increases, more tropical areas are cleared for farmland. Awareness of this problem has done much in recent years to help halt disease.

Flagellum, to help bacterium move

Cytoplasm

Some bacteria have a protective coat

Most bacteria have a rigid cell wall

Nucleoid, containing genetic matter

Bacillus (rod-shaped bacterium)

Hair-like pili anchor bacterium to other cells

NEW TOWNS
This town lies in the heart of the Brazilian rainforest, in South America. Various towns and cities have been built in clearings cut in rainforest. Such towns have suffered many problems. For example, insect-borne disease is common in tropical forests. In order to prevent disease, pools of stagnant water where dangerous insects breed have to be drained. Any scrub where they may rest during the day must be cleared. When planning a new city, the life-cycles of any local disease-causing insects must be considered.

INSIDE A BACTERIUM
A bacterium is a complete living cell, unlike a virus. Some bacteria cause disease by releasing toxins into the body. Others directly invade our cells. Different types target specific kinds of body cells. Bacteria can also change their genetic make-up. This often means that drugs that once combatted the bacteria may no longer work against them.

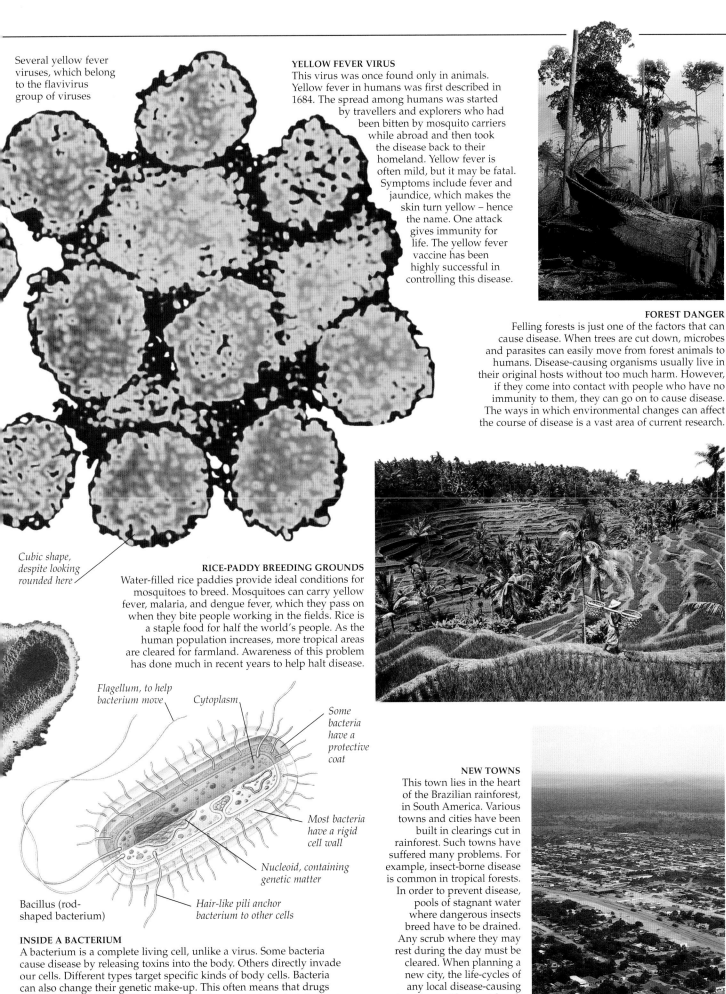

Continental spread

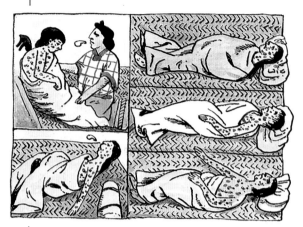

SMALLPOX IN MEXICO
This scene, taken from an old Mexican document, shows native people suffering from smallpox. When the Spanish colonized Mexico, in the 1500s, they brought smallpox with them. By 1521, half the native population was dead and the great civilizations of the Aztec, Maya, and Inca people fell easily to the European invaders.

LONG AGO, PEOPLE TENDED to stay in one area, or migrate slowly when the population became too large. Once the Roman Empire started to spread across the world, around 200 BC, things changed forever. People began to travel more freely, and traded with nomads bringing silk and spices from Asia. When these merchants came home, they brought diseases such as the plague with them that Europeans had never met before, and for which they had no immunity. The same thing happened when Europeans made their way to new lands. The great voyages of exploration in the 1300s and 1400s spread European diseases like measles to vulnerable peoples such as Pacific islanders. Today, travel has become an everyday thing. Thanks to aeroplanes, we can cross the world in a matter of hours – and so can disease. Disease experts know that they must always take travel patterns into account when trying to unravel the course of any new outbreaks.

In the 1500s, it was thought that this arrangement of the planets had caused an outbreak of plague in 1484

Fifteenth-century print by Albrecht Dürer

Syphilis sores

GLOBAL PROBLEMS
This man has fallen prey to syphilis, a once-fatal sexually transmitted disease. The globe deals with an outbreak of plague. Syphilis was common from the 1500s to the 1800s, and the plague raged through much of the world from the 1300s to 1600s. Soldiers and explorers played a huge role in spreading both diseases.

COLUMBUS AND THE AMERICAS
Italian explorer Christopher Columbus and his men first set foot in the Americas in the 1490s, as depicted in this 19th-century print. These men carried diseases such as smallpox and measles, which they passed on to the Native Americans. Those that were weakened by disease were often enslaved and whole populations died.

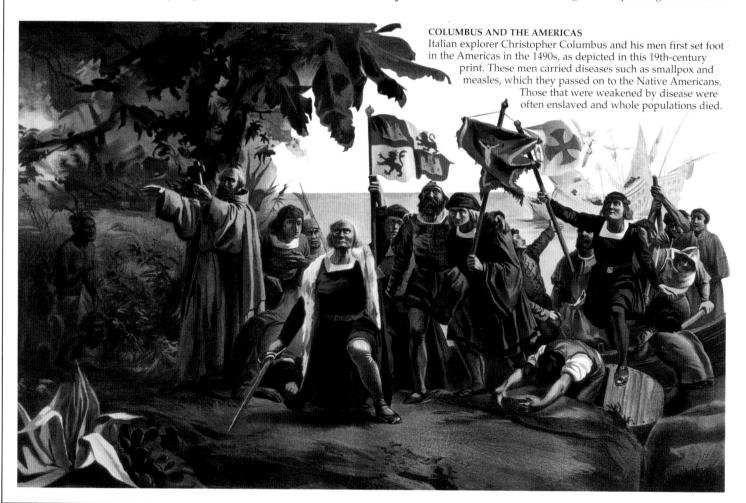

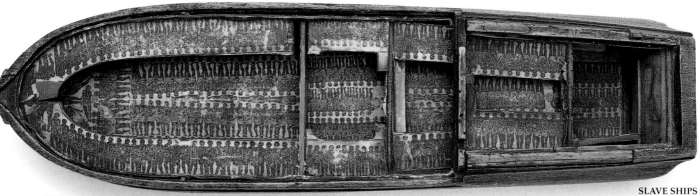

SLAVE SHIPS
This is the kind of ship used to transport black Africans during the days of the slave trade. This trade reached a height around 1800 but ended shortly afterwards. Wealthy Europeans who owned huge cotton and sugar plantations in America and the Caribbean shipped out thousands of slaves from Africa to work on them. In these cramped, unsanitary ships, many died. Survivors often took diseases like yellow fever from Africa to the plantations for which they were bound.

Seventeenth-century fumigating torch

KEEPING THE PLAGUE AWAY
In the 17th century, torches like this were carried to protect against the plague. They were filled with burning aromatic herbs. People at the time believed, wrongly, that the plague was spread by foul odours. They thought that these fumes would keep it away.

Metal "cautery" tool, which was heated and used to burn away the sores suffered by people infected with the plague

Sago from Southeast Asia being loaded onto barges in England, in 1922

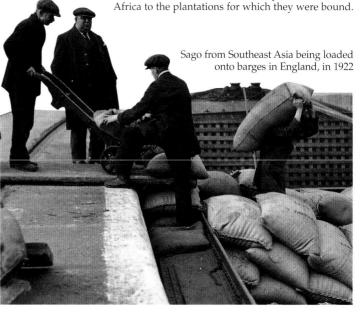

IMPORTED GOODS AND DISEASE
Transporting foods around the world has also helped to spread disease. As transportation has improved, bringing foodstuffs from farther afield, the potential health risk has increased. Moist foodstuffs may be contaminated by disease organisms carried in water. Even a dry food such as rice can occasionally carry diarrhoea-causing microbes. Disease-carrying rats, mice, and insects can easily hide among the cargo in a ship. In many countries, strict health laws control the conditions under which food is brought in from abroad.

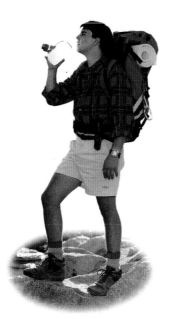

BACKPACKING THE WORLD
Modern transport makes it increasingly easy to reach remote parts of the world, and to come into contact with all kinds of diseases. Some of these take a while to develop. The traveller may return home feeling healthy, but fall ill some weeks later. All travellers should take precautions such as protecting against insect bites, avoiding drinking untreated water, and getting vaccinated.

TAKING TO THE SKIES
Air travel means that a person suffering from a disease can travel thousands of miles in a few hours. This spreads disease to another continent far faster than was possible in the days when people travelled by ship. "Airport malaria" is now a recognized health hazard. The malarial mosquitoes are carried on an aircraft to a destination where the disease never occurs naturally.

Worldwide air travel can spread disease very rapidly

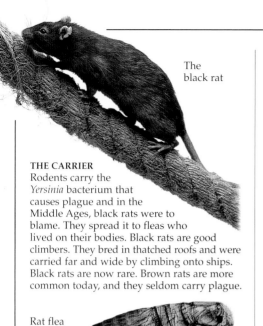

The black rat

The plague

IN THE MIDDLE AGES, THE PLAGUE was one of the most feared diseases. At this time, it was called the Black Death. Starting in the 1300s, epidemics of plague swept the Middle East and Europe, killing up to half the population in some European countries. "Bubonic" plague usually spreads via the bite of infected rat fleas. It causes swollen glands (buboes) in the neck, armpits, and groin. "Pneumonic" plague (affecting the lungs) may also develop, which spreads rapidly by coughing.

Isolated outbreaks continue today in some areas, but it can now be treated with antibiotics. The main part of these pages deals with two great pandemics that hit the world between the 1200s and the 1800s.

THE CARRIER
Rodents carry the *Yersinia* bacterium that causes plague and in the Middle Ages, black rats were to blame. They spread it to fleas who lived on their bodies. Black rats are good climbers. They bred in thatched roofs and were carried far and wide by climbing onto ships. Black rats are now rare. Brown rats are more common today, and they seldom carry plague.

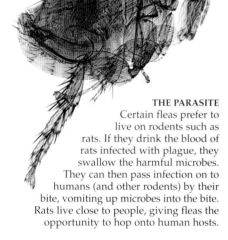

Rat flea

THE PARASITE
Certain fleas prefer to live on rodents such as rats. If they drink the blood of rats infected with plague, they swallow the harmful microbes. They can then pass infection on to humans (and other rodents) by their bite, vomiting up microbes into the bite. Rats live close to people, giving fleas the opportunity to hop onto human hosts.

The Pied Piper lured rats with his pipe-playing

1200s: EARLY SIGNS OF THE BLACK DEATH
It is thought that the medieval outbreak of the Black Death started life in the Himalayas in the 1200s. The legend of the Pied Piper of Hamelin dates from the late 1200s and may be linked with the plague. In the story, the piper rids the German town of Hamelin of rats and then makes its children disappear. This could refer to rats and children dying from the plague.

1300s: EUROPE GRIPPED BY PLAGUE
By 1347, the plague had hit Constantinople (now Istanbul, in Turkey). This was the world's major trading centre and merchants leaving here took the disease all over Europe. It spread rapidly in the cramped, unsanitary conditions of medieval Europe. In some places, people abandoned their homes, and some communities totally died out.

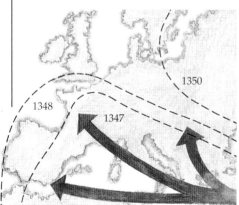

1350

1348

1347

THE PATH OF THE BLACK DEATH
In the 1300s, the Black Death spread from Asia to Europe as Mongol soldiers invaded the West, bringing plague with them. Plague was also brought to Europe by soldiers returning from the Crusades (religious wars against the Muslims) in the Middle East.

Below: summary of major plague dates from ancient times to the present day

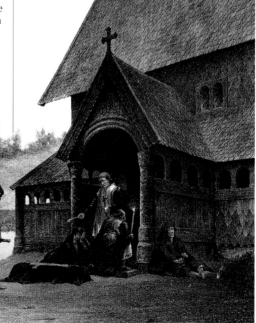

AD 542	AD 610	AD 1330	AD 1347	AD 1665
Justinian's plague (named after an emperor of the time) began in Egypt. The first known pandemic.	Plague reaches China, having travelled from the Middle East, through Persia (now Iran) and India.	Attacking Mongol armies begin their migration to the West. They take the plague with them.	The second pandemic of plague, the Black Death, starts to sweep across the Middle East and Europe.	The Great Plague strikes London. This is stopped by the Great Fire of London, a year later.

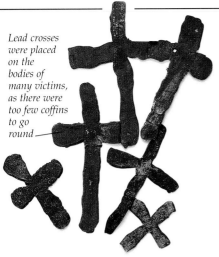

Lead crosses were placed on the bodies of many victims, as there were too few coffins to go round

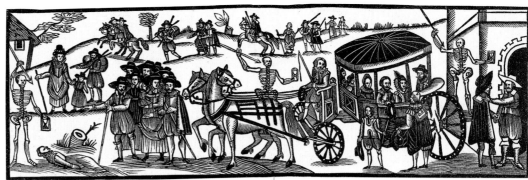

1400s: THE PLAGUE RETURNS
After the first huge wave of deaths in Europe during the mid-1300s, the disease faded and returned every few years. This probably depended on how many rats there were around to spread infection. Generally, these outbreaks were not as severe. In 1479, however, all of England was overwhelmed with plague once more. This time, it killed as many as one person in every five.

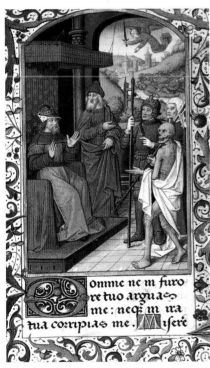

1500s: TEMPORARY RESPITE
By the 1500s, the population of some countries had recovered to their pre-Black Death levels. However, the plague was still a very real threat, as this manuscript illustration shows. Here, the figures of Death, War, and Plague are seen threatening a king, reminding him of his mortality. Outbreaks were still occurring in the 1500s, and they caused many deaths, but they were now less frequent than before.

1600s: FLEEING THE TERROR
In 1665, the Great Plague struck London. Royalty and wealthy people did what many had done before when faced with the plague – they fled the city for the country (the picture above dates from the 1630s). Sadly, this did not help. No one suspected the rats that ran about freely in towns and villages, but they still carried infected fleas. Another disaster followed in 1666, when a huge fire swept through London. However, this burnt down many infected buildings in its wake and brought this major plague outbreak to a halt.

Silver "book" pomander from around 1700. Pomanders like this were carried in a futile attempt to ward off the plague.

Rat image suggests link with the plague

Perforated and filled with fragrant herbs

1700s: KEEPING THE PLAGUE AT BAY
During the 1700s, outbreaks continued, notably in Austria and the Middle East. It was around this time that people carried pomanders like the one above. As it was thought that the plague was caused by foul air, they believed that fragrant fumes would keep it away. Many also sought the advice of unscrupulous "doctors", who sold all kinds of bogus cures.

Quack plague "doctor", 1700s

Elaborate anti-plague mask

1800s: NEW ADVANCES
Various serious outbreaks occurred this century. A huge pandemic began in China, killing 20 million over 75 years. However, the bacterium that causes plague was identified in 1894, and a vaccine developed in 1896.

AD 1721	AD 1855	AD 1900	AD 1960s and 1970s	AD 1994
The second great pandemic finally fades out, in France. However, plague continues in the Middle East.	Third great plague pandemic starts in China. In 1890s, the bacterium is isolated and a vaccine is developed.	A nine-year outbreak of plague hits Sydney and San Francisco, USA. It fades when many rats are killed.	Vietnam becomes the world's leading trouble spot for plague, especially during its war with USA.	Pneumonic plague epidemic breaks out in Surat, India. It kills around 800 people.

Fighting infection

Each day, the body meets millions of harmful microbes, but its powerful immune system can usually deal with them. Invaders have proteins on their surface called antigens. Whenever the immune system does not recognize these, it attacks immediately. If the immune system recognizes them, because it has met these invaders before, an even more effective attack can be launched. In a typical attack, substances called antibodies destroy the microbes, while other cells eat them up. When people are immunized, they are given microbes in a form that makes the immune system respond, but without causing the disease.

LOUIS PASTEUR AND IMMUNIZATION
French chemist Louis Pasteur (1822–1895) discovered that diseases were caused by tiny organisms. In one famous experiment, he showed that animals immunized (vaccinated) with modified anthrax bacteria were protected against catching the disease. Pasteur went on to develop a rabies vaccine. In 1890, he used this to save the life of a boy bitten by a rabid dog.

White blood cell called a macrophage

Shigella bacterium

1 ENGULFING THE ENEMY
The macrophage sends out a projection to engulf a harmful *Shigella* bacterium.

Tiny glass lens

EARLY MICROSCOPES
The first microscopes appeared around 1600. This example was made by Anthoni van Leeuwenhoek (1632–1723). Through his powerful lenses, Leeuwenhoek observed the then-mysterious world of micro-organisms. He gave the first complete descriptions of disease-causing organisms such as bacteria and protozoa, so advancing the study of disease. Much of his work is explained in surviving documents (see below).

Model of microscope designed by Leeuwenhoek

Focusing screw

Collection of Leeuwenhoek's writings, 1695

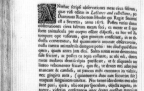

Part of destroyed bacteria on surface of macrophage

2 RECOGNIZING ANTIGENS
A helper T-cell recognizes the particle of destroyed bacteria – antigen – on the surface of the macrophage.

T-cell recognizes antigen and sends chemical messages about it to the B-cell

Helper T-cell (named after the fact that it comes from the thymus gland)

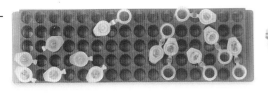

TESTING FOR INFECTION – THE ELISA TEST
The ELISA test is a way of discovering whether a person has antibodies to a specific disease. First, blood plasma (blood with the red cells removed) from the person is stored in a tray like the one above. Samples of the antigens produced by different diseases are then placed in another type of tray. The plasma is dripped onto each antigen sample. A sample changes colour if that antigen reacts with antibodies present in the blood.

PROTECTIVE BUBBLE
Some children have a rare immune disorder. They have to be placed inside a protective plastic bubble and perhaps a sealed suit. This is because their immune systems have not developed correctly early in life, leaving them open to infection. Air entering the bubble is filtered and sterilized to remove microbes. This provides an opportunity for the immune system to develop properly.

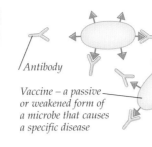

Antibody

Vaccine – a passive or weakened form of a microbe that causes a specific disease

RECEIVING A VACCINATION
The most common way of protecting people against a disease is to give them a type of immunization called a vaccination. Vaccines are often injected into the arm. The body then produces antibodies to fight this particular disease.

Harmful microbe

Antibody

Destroyed organism

HOW VACCINES PROTECT THE BODY
The immune system "remembers" the antibodies produced by the vaccine. If the same harmful microbe invades in the future, the immune system recognizes and destroys it. Protection from a vaccine may last weeks, months, years, or for a lifetime.

Device for dripping plasma onto antigen samples

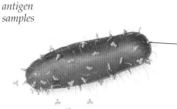

Antibodies attach themselves to Shigella bacteria

5 TAGGING THE BACTERIA
The antibodies "tag" the *Shigella* bacteria, so that the immune system recognizes and destroys this specific type of bacteria.

HOW THE IMMUNE SYSTEM FIGHTS INFECTION
The immune system works in a cycle. The main players are white cells found in the immune system: macrophages, T-cells, and B-cells. A macrophage destroys a bacterium or a cluster of viruses. Bits of protein (antigens) from the microbes move to the surface of the macrophage, where they can be recognized by the immune system. Helper T-cells send messages to B-cells, which change into cells producing antibodies against the antigen.

Lymph nodes – dense lymph tissue containing a cluster of white cells. The nodes filter lymph as part of its circulation around the body

Antibody

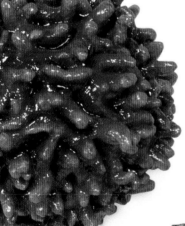

B-cell

3 RECEIVING THE MESSAGE
The B-cell recognizes chemical messages from the T-cell. The B-cell multiplies and some of the new cells turn into plasma cells.

4 RELEASING ANTIBODIES
The plasma cells release antibodies to fight *Shigella* bacteria (shown above right).

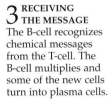

Plasma cell

The main lymph-carrying vessels are called lymphatics; finer ones are called lymph capillaries

THE LYMPH SYSTEM
The human immune system consists of the lymph system and organs such as the thymus. The thymus controls production of the white blood cells that fight infection (which start life in the bone marrow). The lymph system is a series of channels running right around the body. Through these channels flows lymph – a colourless liquid that originates in the bloodstream. Lymph contains white cells such as T- and B-cells.

Epidemics and the city

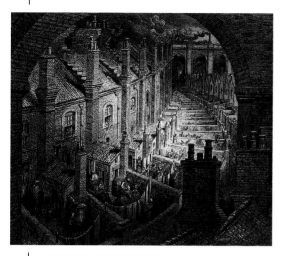

WHEN PEOPLE LIVED IN small farming groups, disease seldom spread very far. As towns and cities grew up, epidemics started to break out. People crowded together in filthy conditions – the ideal way to spread microbes. No one knew what caused disease, so town- and city-dwellers rarely washed, handled dirty food, and drank water contaminated with human waste. In some of the world's major cities, the Industrial Revolution of the 1700s and 1800s brought vast expansion. By the 19th century, diseases such as typhoid killed hundreds every year in London and New York. These diseases are still a problem in countries that are too poor to control them.

THE CITY AND INDUSTRY
This 19th-century engraving shows what much of London looked like at the height of the Industrial Revolution. The 1800s was the great era of mechanization and manufacturing. People flooded into cities to find work in factories, mines, railways, and shops. Narrow streets were filled with smoke and rubbish. Workers lived crammed together in tiny homes with no running water and poor sanitation.

SCREENING AT ELLIS ISLAND
Here, immigrant children arriving in the USA are checked over and screened for diseases such as typhoid and cholera. Between 1892 and 1954, people entering the USA from abroad were given a full examination. This took place at Ellis Island, New York. The sick were refused entry and kept in isolation.

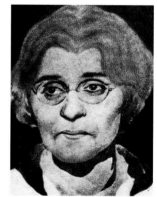

"Typhoid Mary"

TYPHOID MARY
Mary Mallon was a cook in New York. She earned her nickname by infecting at least 53 people with typhoid between 1900 and 1915. Working as a cook, she spread the disease by handling food. She herself had recovered from the disease but became a carrier (live bacteria lived in her body though she showed no signs of illness). Because she refused to stop working as a cook, she was confined to an isolation hospital.

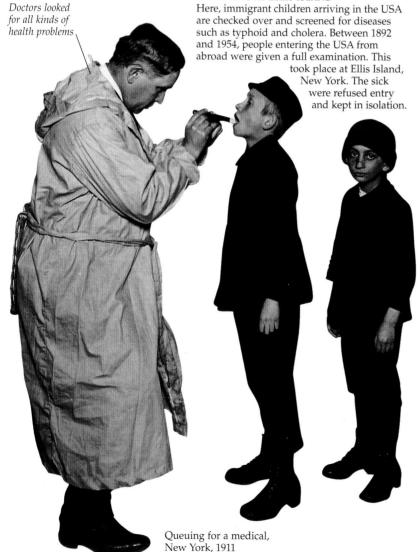

Doctors looked for all kinds of health problems

Queuing for a medical, New York, 1911

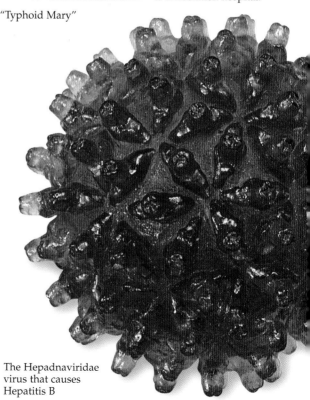

The Hepadnaviridae virus that causes Hepatitis B

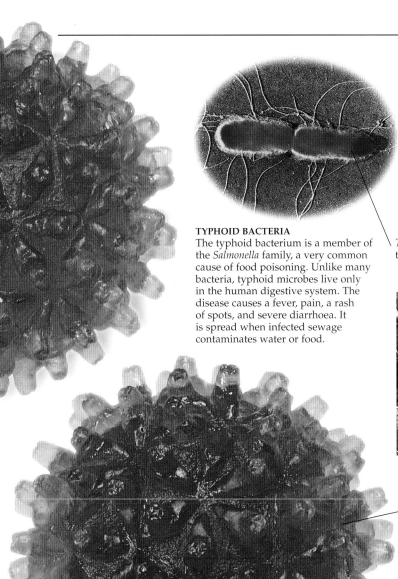

TYPHOID BACTERIA
The typhoid bacterium is a member of the *Salmonella* family, a very common cause of food poisoning. Unlike many bacteria, typhoid microbes live only in the human digestive system. The disease causes a fever, pain, a rash of spots, and severe diarrhoea. It is spread when infected sewage contaminates water or food.

CONTAMINATED WATER
A town or city needs a huge supply of drinking water. This must be free of microbes to stop the diseases that spread rapidly when people are crammed together. In some countries, the same water is used for a variety of different purposes, and this can spread disease. The standard of water supplies in cities has improved dramatically over the last 100 years. Aid organizations always make this a priority, wherever they are working.

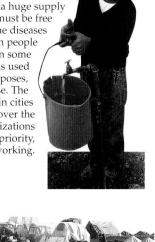

The rod-shaped Salmonella typhi *bacteria that cause typhoid*

The hepatitis virus targets the body's liver cells

REFUGEE CAMPS
Other large settlements, such as refugee camps, suffer many of the same problems as cities. People end up living in crowded temporary camps when war causes them to flee their homes. They are often starving when they arrive, making them vulnerable to disease. Typhoid, typhus, and cholera almost always accompany such camps. It is a race to vaccinate people and provide adequate shelter, water, food, and sanitation before disease strikes.

DISCARDED NEEDLES
Used, discarded needles are a danger in many cities, where needle-borne diseases such as hepatitis B thrive. The hepatitis B virus, for example, can survive outside the body for a year. Needles must be disposed of carefully to prevent people from accidentally handling them. Drug addicts often use needles repeatedly or share them. Distributing once-only, disposable syringes has helped. However, these may also be shared and their design makes them difficult to clean properly.

HEPATITIS B VIRUS
The virus that causes hepatitis B is transmitted by sexual contact and infected blood. Like HIV, this disease is common among drug abusers who share needles, but is far more infectious. Fever, jaundice, and sickness are common symptoms. Hepatitis means inflammation of the liver and comes in various forms. The types caused by viruses are called hepatitis A, B, and C. Hepatitis A is spread by contaminated food and water. Hepatitis C usually originates with infected blood.

For hepatitis B, three vaccines like this are given over a period of six months

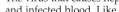

HEPATITIS B VACCINE
People likely to be exposed to hepatitis B can now receive a vaccine to protect them from the infection. Vaccination is usually recommended for people such as doctors and police officers, who may come into contact with infected blood during their normal work. There are not yet effective vaccines for all types of hepatitis, only against hepatitis B and hepatitis A.

Food poisoning

WHEN PEOPLE TALK ABOUT FOOD POISONING, they usually mean one of several common bacterial infections caught from eating contaminated food. Likely culprits include the bacteria *Salmonella* and *E. coli* (*Escheriscia coli*). Symptoms vary from a mild stomach upset to cramps, vomiting, and diarrhoea. This can be serious if it goes on for too long, as the body loses a lot of water and valuable tissue salts. *Salmonella* and *E. coli* are commonly found existing harmlessly in farm animals, but may cause illness when passed on to us in foods such as meat and eggs – especially if they have not been cooked well enough to kill the bacteria. Listeriosis is another bacterial disease. It may come from animals, although this bacteria also harms their health in various ways. Our immune system can learn to deal with certain bacteria, but will still be vulnerable to related forms.

Flagellae allow E. coli to move more quickly

Cilia help bacteria to stick to intestinal wall

Rod-like shape

E. COLI
We encounter both harmless and harmful kinds of *E. coli* all the time. Harmless *E. coli* live permanently in our digestive system, helping to keep it in a healthy, balanced state. We become immune to harmful forms that we meet regularly, but will still be vulnerable to other dangerous strains.

How *E. coli* 0157:H7 attacks the intestines

Special proteins and hairs on the surface of the bacteria help it stick to the intestines

HOW *E. COLI* ATTACKS THE BODY
Potentially harmful *E. coli* bacteria, including the type 0157:H7 (below), enter the body through the mouth and make their way to the intestines. They have special surface proteins that allow them to stick firmly to the intestine wall without being carried away by food passing through the digestive system. *E. coli* such as 0157:H7 also secrete poisons that damage the cells lining the intestines. These damaged cells eventually die and pass out of the body, producing bloody diarrhoea.

Mucus cells in intestine wall. Mucus makes the wall slimy, but the E. coli are still able to cling on.

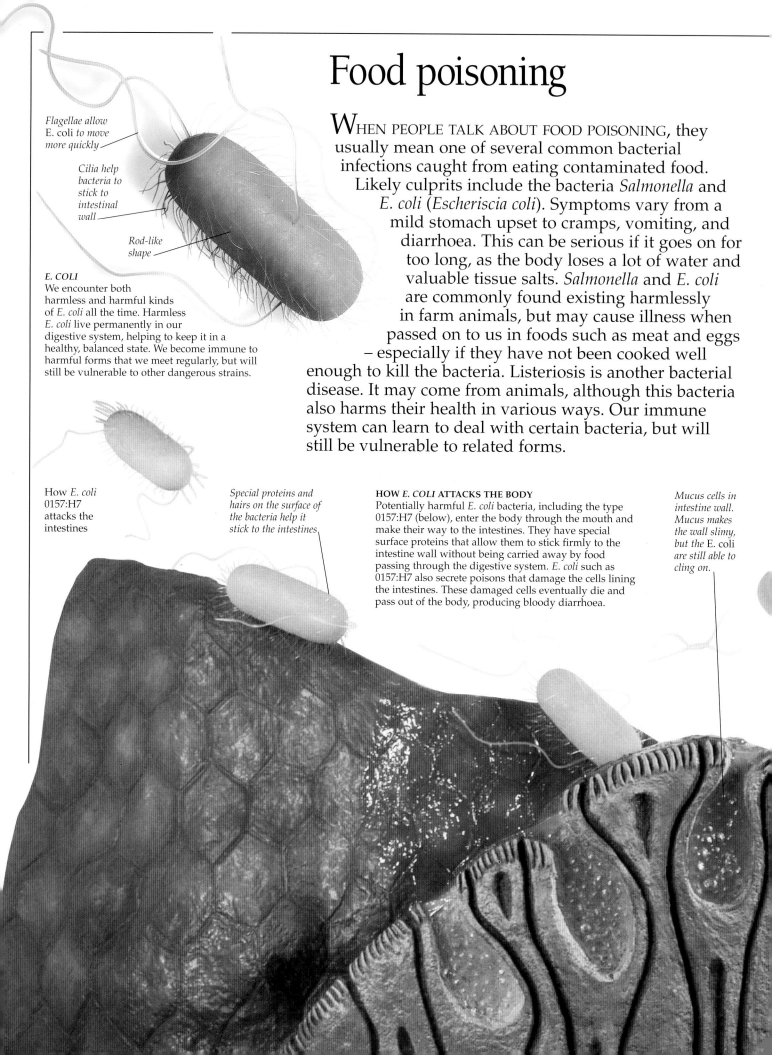

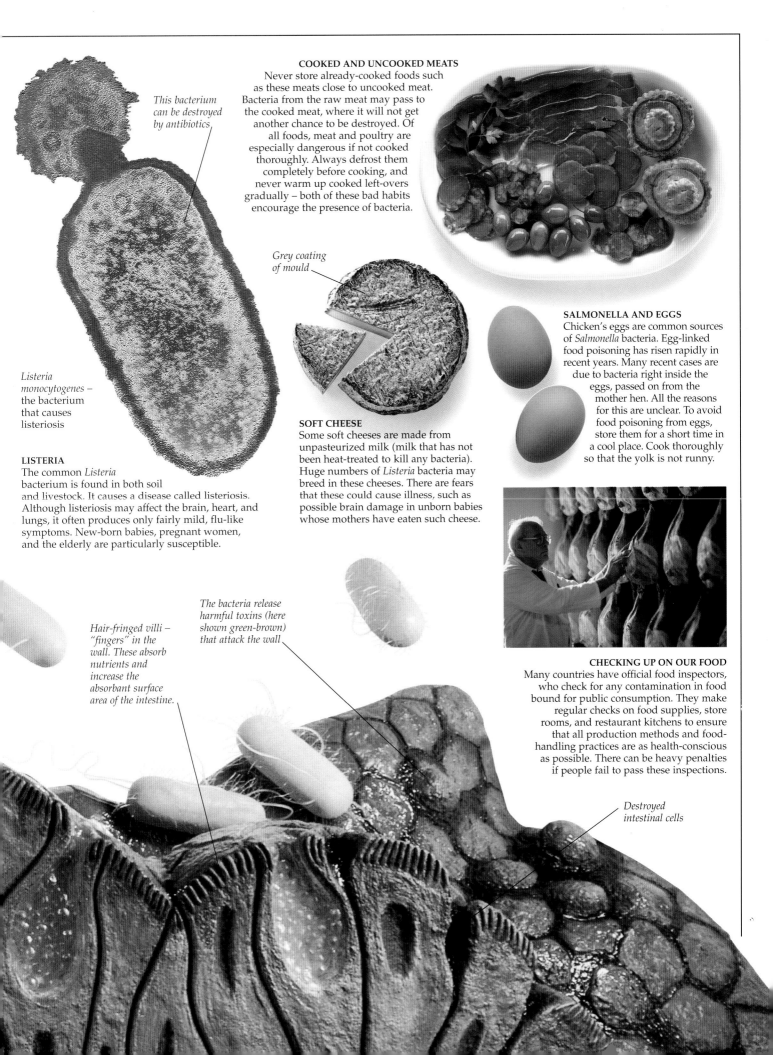

COOKED AND UNCOOKED MEATS
Never store already-cooked foods such as these meats close to uncooked meat. Bacteria from the raw meat may pass to the cooked meat, where it will not get another chance to be destroyed. Of all foods, meat and poultry are especially dangerous if not cooked thoroughly. Always defrost them completely before cooking, and never warm up cooked left-overs gradually – both of these bad habits encourage the presence of bacteria.

This bacterium can be destroyed by antibiotics

Grey coating of mould

Listeria monocytogenes – the bacterium that causes listeriosis

LISTERIA
The common *Listeria* bacterium is found in both soil and livestock. It causes a disease called listeriosis. Although listeriosis may affect the brain, heart, and lungs, it often produces only fairly mild, flu-like symptoms. New-born babies, pregnant women, and the elderly are particularly susceptible.

SOFT CHEESE
Some soft cheeses are made from unpasteurized milk (milk that has not been heat-treated to kill any bacteria). Huge numbers of *Listeria* bacteria may breed in these cheeses. There are fears that these could cause illness, such as possible brain damage in unborn babies whose mothers have eaten such cheese.

SALMONELLA AND EGGS
Chicken's eggs are common sources of *Salmonella* bacteria. Egg-linked food poisoning has risen rapidly in recent years. Many recent cases are due to bacteria right inside the eggs, passed on from the mother hen. All the reasons for this are unclear. To avoid food poisoning from eggs, store them for a short time in a cool place. Cook thoroughly so that the yolk is not runny.

CHECKING UP ON OUR FOOD
Many countries have official food inspectors, who check for any contamination in food bound for public consumption. They make regular checks on food supplies, store rooms, and restaurant kitchens to ensure that all production methods and food-handling practices are as health-conscious as possible. There can be heavy penalties if people fail to pass these inspections.

Hair-fringed villi – "fingers" in the wall. These absorb nutrients and increase the absorbant surface area of the intestine.

The bacteria release harmful toxins (here shown green-brown) that attack the wall

Destroyed intestinal cells

Water and raw foods

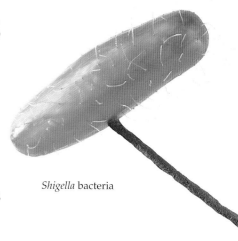

CONTAMINATED DRINKING WATER is a major cause of sickness and diarrhoea. If disease-carrying water is used to wash foods such as salads, which are not cooked to destroy microbes, then this too can lead to problems. Contamination of water and uncooked food often comes from microbes in human waste, so hygiene plays a huge role. Microbes love dirty, crowded places with no proper sanitation and spread rapidly when food-handlers do not wash their hands. Major microbes thriving in these kinds of conditions include *Giardia* protozoa and *Shigella* bacteria. *Giardia* is often found in the intestines doing no damage at all, but it can also cause unpleasant diarrhoea, while *Shigella* can produce a serious illness called dysentery.

Shigella bacteria

GERM-CARRIER
The common housefly is responsible for a great deal of bacterial food contamination, thanks to its feeding habits. Flies are attracted to dead and decaying matter, including human waste. Picking up bacteria as they walk over infected material, they then transfer it to any piece of food, crockery, or cutlery that they might land on.

Flies spread germs by walking over cutlery, crockery, and food

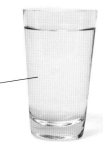

A glass of tap water can be risky in some parts of the world, so take only bottled water if in doubt – even for cleaning your teeth

COMMON PROBLEM FOODS
Raw foods such as fruit and salads may harbour microbes that have not been destroyed by cooking. Rinsing them in water can make matters worse if the water itself is contaminated. The problem is most acute in parts of the world where warm, humid temperatures encourage disease to flourish and where sanitation standards are poor. In these places, avoid salads and peel fruit before eating it.

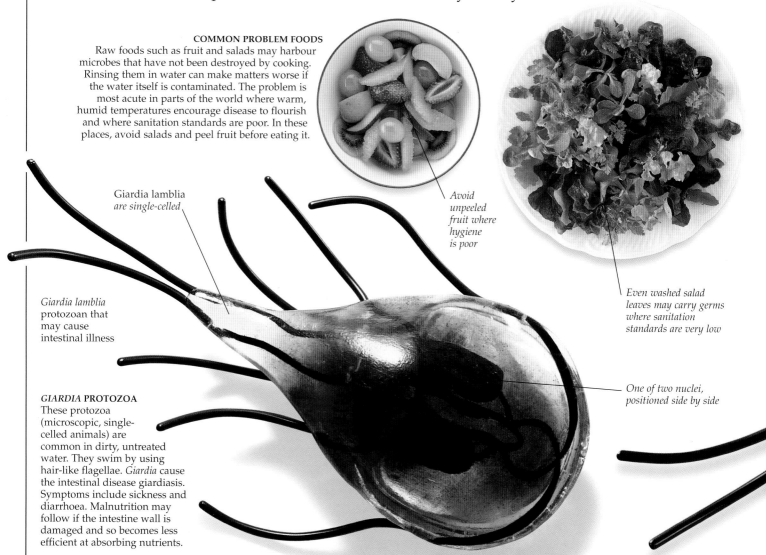

Avoid unpeeled fruit where hygiene is poor

Even washed salad leaves may carry germs where sanitation standards are very low

Giardia lamblia *are single-celled*

Giardia lamblia *protozoan that may cause intestinal illness*

One of two nuclei, positioned side by side

***GIARDIA* PROTOZOA**
These protozoa (microscopic, single-celled animals) are common in dirty, untreated water. They swim by using hair-like flagellae. *Giardia* cause the intestinal disease giardiasis. Symptoms include sickness and diarrhoea. Malnutrition may follow if the intestine wall is damaged and so becomes less efficient at absorbing nutrients.

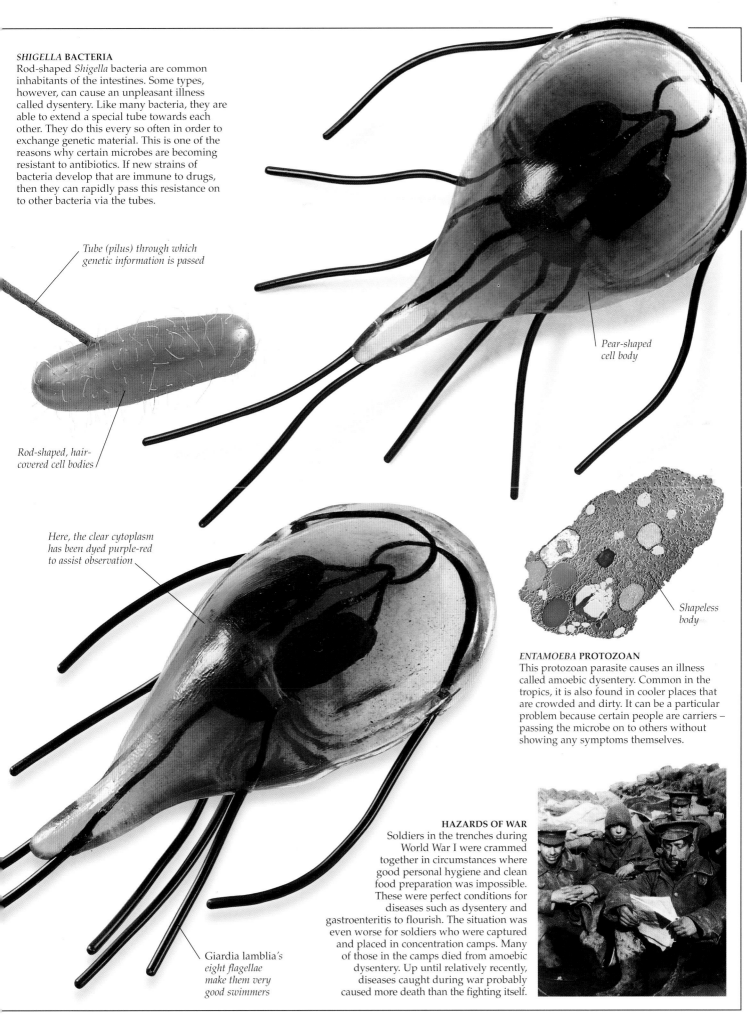

SHIGELLA BACTERIA

Rod-shaped *Shigella* bacteria are common inhabitants of the intestines. Some types, however, can cause an unpleasant illness called dysentery. Like many bacteria, they are able to extend a special tube towards each other. They do this every so often in order to exchange genetic material. This is one of the reasons why certain microbes are becoming resistant to antibiotics. If new strains of bacteria develop that are immune to drugs, then they can rapidly pass this resistance on to other bacteria via the tubes.

Tube (pilus) through which genetic information is passed

Rod-shaped, hair-covered cell bodies

Here, the clear cytoplasm has been dyed purple-red to assist observation

Pear-shaped cell body

Shapeless body

ENTAMOEBA PROTOZOAN

This protozoan parasite causes an illness called amoebic dysentery. Common in the tropics, it is also found in cooler places that are crowded and dirty. It can be a particular problem because certain people are carriers – passing the microbe on to others without showing any symptoms themselves.

Giardia lamblia's eight flagellae make them very good swimmers

HAZARDS OF WAR

Soldiers in the trenches during World War I were crammed together in circumstances where good personal hygiene and clean food preparation was impossible. These were perfect conditions for diseases such as dysentery and gastroenteritis to flourish. The situation was even worse for soldiers who were captured and placed in concentration camps. Many of those in the camps died from amoebic dysentery. Up until relatively recently, diseases caught during war probably caused more death than the fighting itself.

Cholera

A WATERBORNE DISEASE, cholera occurs when water supplies are contaminated by the bacterium *Vibrio cholerae*. Once swallowed, the bacteria multiply in the intestines and release toxins. Symptoms include vomiting and diarrhoea, which may lead to the body losing large amounts of fluid and vital body salts. The first major cholera epidemic occurred in India in the early 1800s. Sailors and traders visiting the area picked up the disease and carried it rapidly around the world by ship. It soon spread to Asia and the Middle East, reaching Europe and the USA in 1832. By the end of the 19th century, however, improved sanitation had freed Europe and North America from the disease. The importance of fresh water and proper sanitation was realized after an outbreak in London, in 1854. A certain Dr Snow traced the outbreak to a public drinking water pump in Broad Street. Water here was contaminated by a faulty sewer pipe. Once the pump was closed, the cholera stopped.

CHOLERA THE KILLER
A contemporary illustration of the Balkan Wars of 1912 shows Death scything down troops during a cholera epidemic. Cholera can be a devastating killer because it appears suddenly and spreads quickly. Today, although no long-term vaccine exists, we are much more aware of drinking clean water and so can take effective steps to prevent the disease from gaining a hold in the first place.

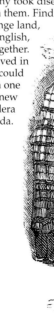

BOUND FOR AMERICA
Many immigrants travelled from Europe to North America during the 1800s and 1900s. Most were poor people who went in search of a better life. Many took diseases such as cholera with them. Finding themselves in a strange land, often unable to speak English, the migrants clustered together. With little money, they lived in slums. Here, disease could spread very rapidly. In one month alone, 1,220 new arrivals died of cholera in Montreal, Canada.

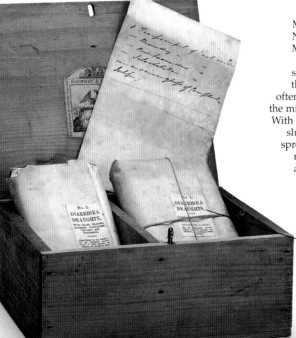

Opium-based medicine to ease pain

"Anti-cholera" medicine chest from the 1800s

Medicine to soothe the inflamed intestines

CHOLERA CHEST
Nineteenth-century travellers often carried medicine chests like this. They contained drugs to alleviate cholera, including the powerful painkiller, opium. Drinking plenty of sweet drinks, such as iced lemon and barley water, helped the patient to recover from fluid-loss. In 1893, the modern vaccine was developed. This gives some protection from infection, but only for a short time.

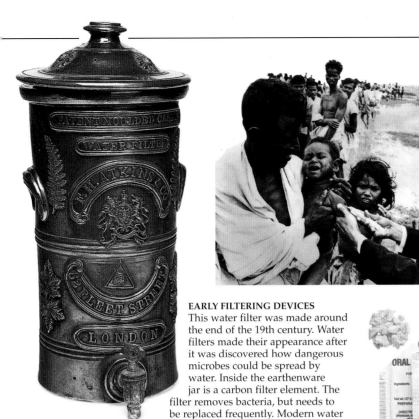

NATURAL DISASTERS
Here, World Health Organization workers react rapidly to give a short-term vaccination to those at risk after a cyclone strikes India and Bangladesh. Cholera is often a threat after a natural disaster. The fierce winds of a cyclone, for example, cause tides to push back coastal waters. Rivers flood vast areas of low-lying land, destroying villages and drowning people and animals as they go. In these conditions, cholera quickly takes hold as people are exposed to contaminated or untreated drinking water.

REHYDRATION KIT
A simple kit of powdered medicine and a dosing spoon has saved millions of people across the world from the effects of cholera. The most dangerous symptom is loss of body salts and fluid from sickness and diarrhoea. If a powder containing sodium and potassium salts and sugar is dissolved in clean water and drunk, this will help to get the body back on course. Once rehydrated, the body's immune system is better able to fight infection.

EARLY FILTERING DEVICES
This water filter was made around the end of the 19th century. Water filters made their appearance after it was discovered how dangerous microbes could be spread by water. Inside the earthenware jar is a carbon filter element. The filter removes bacteria, but needs to be replaced frequently. Modern water filters follow the same principle.

Compact dosing "spoon"

The sachets of powder are mixed with water

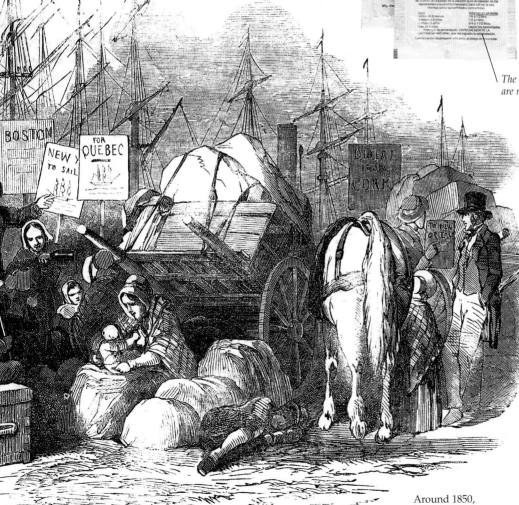

Around 1850, emigrants gather on a quayside in Cork, Ireland before embarking for the USA

CHOLERA TODAY
Some poorer countries still have a cholera problem, especially in the cities. The poor often live in slums where inadequate sanitation contaminates drinking water. Less strict hygiene laws also allow the disease to spread. In Lima, Peru in 1991, ships from India emptied their ballast tanks in the harbour. Thousands of gallons of water were released that contained a cholera bacterium. This contaminated the fish that local people loved to eat and cholera swept through Latin America.

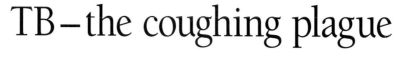

TB – the coughing plague

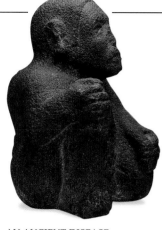

AN ANCIENT DISEASE
This Mexican Aztec sculpture dates from about 500 years ago. It clearly shows the deformed back that is a typical symptom of TB. Tuberculosis has been affecting people for at least 5,000 years. Evidence of tuberculosis infection has also been found in Stone Age skeletons and Egyptian mummies.

TUBERCULOSIS (TB) HAS BEEN WITH US for centuries. Caused by bacteria, it spreads when infected people cough, sneeze, or talk. This releases tiny water droplets filled with microbes that are inhaled by other people. TB thrives in dirty cities where people are crammed together. In the 1700s and 1800s, the world's major industrial cities were in the grip of "consumption", as TB was known. By the early 1900s, better living conditions had brought it under control. In 1922 a vaccine appeared and the first anti-TB drug, streptomycin, was developed in 1944. Widespread pasteurization of milk also helped greatly as this killed the TB bacillus found in cows' milk. Today, TB is still present in crowded areas with poor health care and sanitation, but aid agencies are working hard to combat its spread.

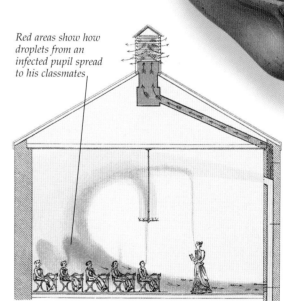

TB TOUCH PIECES
These gold pieces date from the reign of James I (1603–1625) of England. They were used in "touch" ceremonies, where the king bestowed his supposedly healing touch on sick people. People believed that rulers had healing powers because they were granted their position by God. The touch was thought to be especially effective against scrofula, a form of TB that often causes ulcers on the neck.

Red areas show how droplets from an infected pupil spread to his classmates

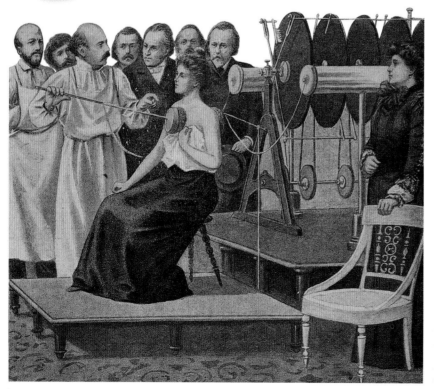

THE IMPORTANCE OF VENTILATION
This diagram of a school was published in 1894. It shows how certain ventilation systems can assist the spread of diseases such as TB, which is carried in the air. Bad, infected air is swept upwards, but not before it has gathered at the bottom of the classroom. It swirls around the pupils, putting them in danger of infection.

QUACK TREATMENTS
In the early 1900s, journals featured all kinds of strange anti-TB devices. This one applied an electrical current to the TB sufferer's chest – it did not work. In past eras, doctors were often helpless in the face of disease and "quack" (false and odd) miracle cures flourished. If the disease progressed slowly, as TB does, patients were often convinced that such treatments were effective.

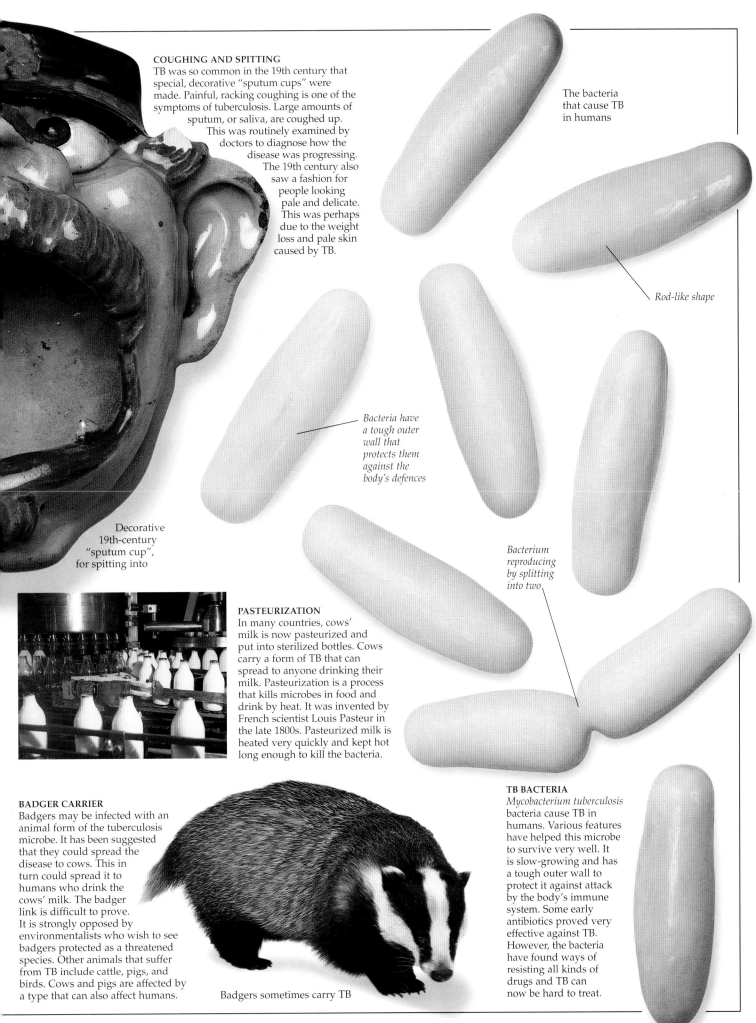

COUGHING AND SPITTING

TB was so common in the 19th century that special, decorative "sputum cups" were made. Painful, racking coughing is one of the symptoms of tuberculosis. Large amounts of sputum, or saliva, are coughed up. This was routinely examined by doctors to diagnose how the disease was progressing. The 19th century also saw a fashion for people looking pale and delicate. This was perhaps due to the weight loss and pale skin caused by TB.

Decorative 19th-century "sputum cup", for spitting into

The bacteria that cause TB in humans

Rod-like shape

Bacteria have a tough outer wall that protects them against the body's defences

Bacterium reproducing by splitting into two

PASTEURIZATION

In many countries, cows' milk is now pasteurized and put into sterilized bottles. Cows carry a form of TB that can spread to anyone drinking their milk. Pasteurization is a process that kills microbes in food and drink by heat. It was invented by French scientist Louis Pasteur in the late 1800s. Pasteurized milk is heated very quickly and kept hot long enough to kill the bacteria.

BADGER CARRIER

Badgers may be infected with an animal form of the tuberculosis microbe. It has been suggested that they could spread the disease to cows. This in turn could spread it to humans who drink the cows' milk. The badger link is difficult to prove. It is strongly opposed by environmentalists who wish to see badgers protected as a threatened species. Other animals that suffer from TB include cattle, pigs, and birds. Cows and pigs are affected by a type that can also affect humans.

Badgers sometimes carry TB

TB BACTERIA

Mycobacterium tuberculosis bacteria cause TB in humans. Various features have helped this microbe to survive very well. It is slow-growing and has a tough outer wall to protect it against attack by the body's immune system. Some early antibiotics proved very effective against TB. However, the bacteria have found ways of resisting all kinds of drugs and TB can now be hard to treat.

Lepers and leprosy

THE MIDDLE AGES saw many terrible epidemics spread across Europe and Asia. One of these was leprosy, thought to be among the oldest of human diseases. This bacterial illness is probably spread via droplets of nasal mucus, but contrary to popular belief is extremely hard to catch. This is partly because the illness is only infectious in its early stages, and only certain people are vulnerable. Leprosy progresses very slowly, attacking the skin and nerves and causing severe facial distortions. Parts of the body become numb and prone to damage. Infection and mutilation often follow and many people lose fingers, toes, ears, and noses. Now rare in the West, the disease affects about six million people worldwide. Most of us carry leprosy antibodies, which means that at some time we have been exposed to the bacterium without becoming ill.

Illuminated (decorated) manuscript depicting St Giles

THE PATRON SAINT OF LEPERS
St Giles, who was originally called Aegidius, lived around AD 700 and later became the patron saint of lepers. For centuries, leprosy was shrouded in mystery, due to its slow progress and terrible mutilations. Shunned by society, and mostly ignored by doctors, lepers could do little for themselves except resort to prayer.

The facial distortions caused by leprosy were said to make sufferers look like lions

Damaged limbs covered up with bandages

Microscope slide of a leprosy sufferer's damaged nerve cells

Medieval leper

Leper "clapper"

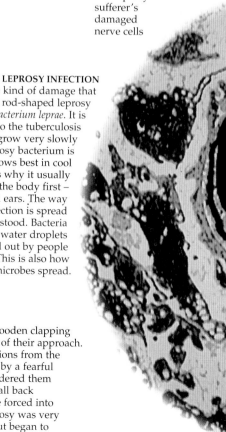

LEPROSY INFECTION
This shows the kind of damage that can be done by the rod-shaped leprosy bacterium, *Mycobacterium leprae*. It is closely related to the tuberculosis bacterium – both grow very slowly in the body. The leprosy bacterium is peculiar because it grows best in cool conditions. This is why it usually strikes cooler parts of the body first – such as fingers and ears. The way in which leprosy infection is spread is not fully understood. Bacteria may well spread in water droplets coughed or sneezed out by people with the disease. This is also how tuberculosis microbes spread.

CAST OUT BY SOCIETY
Medieval lepers had to carry wooden clapping devices or bells to warn people of their approach. They also covered their mutilations from the public's terrified eyes. Cast out by a fearful and ignorant society who considered them "unclean", most lepers had to fall back on a life of begging. Many were forced into special isolation hospitals. Leprosy was very common in the Middle Ages, but began to disappear after the ravages of the Black Death, although no one knows why this was.

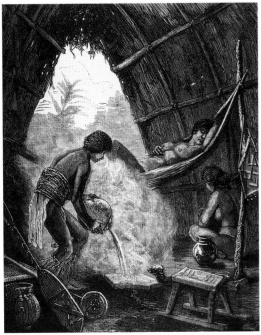

Nineteenth-century print of a traditional South American leprosy cure

HANSEN'S DISEASE
The leprosy bacterium was first described in 1874 by a Norwegian physician called Armauer Hansen (1841–1912). Up until this point, many people had thought that the disease was hereditary. Hansen concluded that leprosy was infectious and showed that it could be controlled partly by isolating sufferers. Leprosy has often been referred to as Hansen's disease, because of the stigma attached to the word "leprosy".

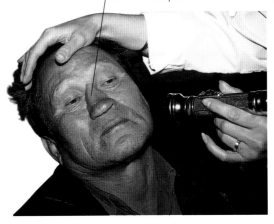

Patient's damaged nose has collapsed

OUTER SIGNS AND SYMPTOMS
This man is showing the early effects of leprosy infection. Bacteria have invaded the cells of his nose. Destruction of the rubbery cartilage that supports the nose has caused it to collapse. Later stages can include ulcers and sores, which may become infected and cause further damage. There are different forms of leprosy, affecting certain areas of the body.

SOUTH AMERICAN STEAM TREATMENT
A steam bath was one of the ways in which native South Americans once tried to ease the pain of leprosy in its early stages. Along with many other diseases, leprosy travelled to North and South America with European explorers and colonizers. It found a large population who had never encountered the leprosy bacteria before. They had no immunity and the disease was able to spread rapidly.

Herbal oil treatment

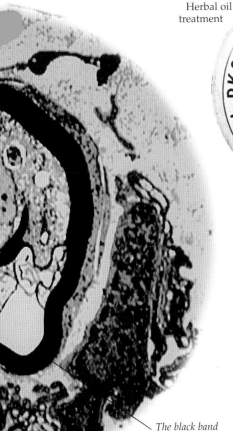

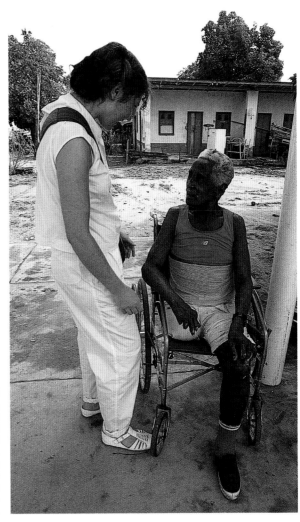

NATURAL RELIEF
Chaulmoogra ointment is a natural, traditional Hindu remedy for leprosy sores. Based on a herbal oil extracted from an Indian tree, it brings some healing pain relief. Modern anti-leprosy drugs work by killing the bacteria. They can produce rapid results if they are used before the disease is well-established.

MODERN LEPROSY HOSPITALS
Specialist leprosy hospitals and clinics, such as this one in Brazil, are found in countries where the disease is still common. Many leprosy sufferers in these hospitals are long-term patients. They need to live in for a while because treatment of more advanced cases is a slow process. Also, many sufferers are so damaged by the infection that they can no longer live independent lives.

The black band is a nerve fibre's protective sheath, seen here breaking up

Outsmarting the smallpox virus

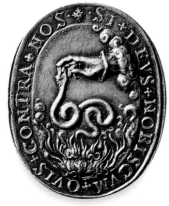

COMMEMORATIVE COIN
Silver coins were struck to give thanks for the survival of Queen Elizabeth I of England after she almost died from smallpox in 1562. Over the years, royalty reflected the high incidence of the disease. Peter II of Russia, Louis XV of France, and Luis I of Spain all died from smallpox.

Smallpox is the only illness to have been wiped out as a human disease. The official announcement of its eradication came in 1980. Caused by a virus, and highly infectious, smallpox produces flu-like symptoms. More serious problems such as kidney failure may follow, and around half of its victims once died. The disease causes pus-filled swellings of the skin that leave pitted scars. Cases were so numerous in the 18th and 19th centuries that few people took any notice of anyone with smallpox scars.

The disease was first described in Roman times. Outbreaks occurred across Europe, Asia, and Africa, and Europeans took it to North and South America. In the 1700s, a safe vaccination was developed and the path to success began.

THE GOD OF SMALLPOX
Yuo-hoa-long was the Chinese god of recovery from smallpox. People begged him for protection, just as people in Europe prayed to Christian saints to keep them from harm. The Chinese were the first to introduce protective measures against smallpox, in AD 590. People were inoculated with pus taken from victims suffering from a mild form of the disease. Some people gained protection, but the practice also led to fresh outbreaks.

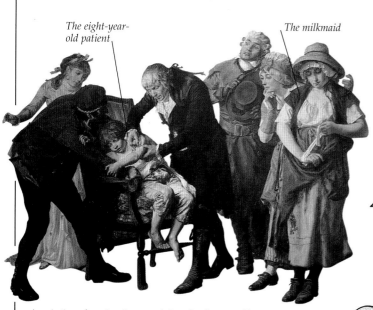

The eight-year-old patient

The milkmaid

A painting showing Jenner giving the first smallpox vaccine

DR EDWARD JENNER
Edward Jenner (1749–1823) was an English doctor. In 1796 he performed the first successful vaccination against smallpox. Jenner noticed that farm workers who caught cowpox (a similar, but mild disease of cattle) never caught smallpox. Jenner vaccinated eight-year-old James Phipps with fluid from a cowpox blister on a milkmaid's hand. Six weeks later, he inoculated the boy with a mild form of smallpox – and no infection developed.

The Chinese god of smallpox, Yuo-hoa-long

JENNER'S COWHORN AND LANCET

Edward Jenner used this lancet to puncture two cuts in his patient James Phipps' arm. The piece of horn below belonged to a cow from which Jenner obtained cowpox virus to use in a vaccination against smallpox. Jenner's technique was widely adopted and deaths from smallpox fell dramatically. The term vaccination was named after the Latin word *vacca*, meaning "cow".

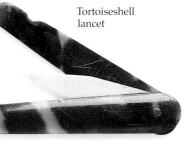

Tortoiseshell lancet

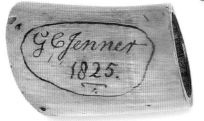

Piece of cow horn

EARLY VACCINATOR

The sharp teeth on this 19th-century vaccinator were used to scratch the skin so that fluid from cowpox sores could enter. This would produce a mild infection of cowpox that gave immunity against smallpox. The device is curved so that it can fit snugly over the arm of a small child.

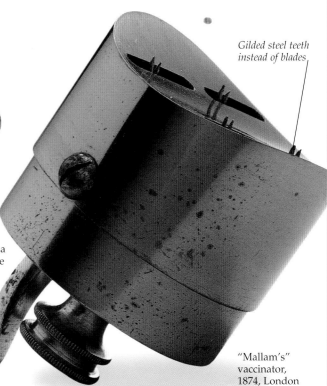

Gilded steel teeth instead of blades

"Mallam's" vaccinator, 1874, London

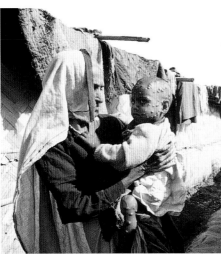

A WORLDWIDE PROGRAMME

A member of the Red Cross aid agency vaccinates a Sudanese child against smallpox. In the 1970s, the World Health Organization, working with international aid and medical agencies, began a campaign to eradicate smallpox. Even in the most remote parts of the world, people were vaccinated wherever smallpox was reported.

THE SMALLPOX VIRUS

This electron micrograph shows the structure of the variola virus that causes smallpox. The green outer layer is a protective protein coat. The red core contains genetic material, which this virus injects into human cells in order to infect them. After smallpox was eradicated, the frozen virus was preserved under heavy guard in a few laboratories around the world for future research. Unlike most potentially fatal diseases, there is no animal reservoir of smallpox, so it can never reappear naturally.

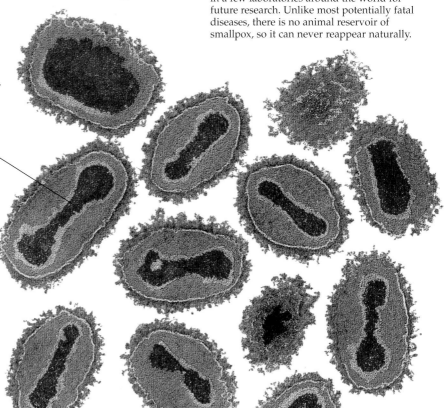

Core of genetic material

The variola virus that causes smallpox

THE LAST SMALLPOX OUTBREAKS

This picture of a child in Bangladesh was taken in 1973. It shows the typical sores caused by smallpox infection. A man in Somalia was the last natural victim of the disease, in 1977. In 1980 the World Health Organization was finally able to declare that smallpox had been eradicated worldwide – an extraordinary achievement.

Raging rabies

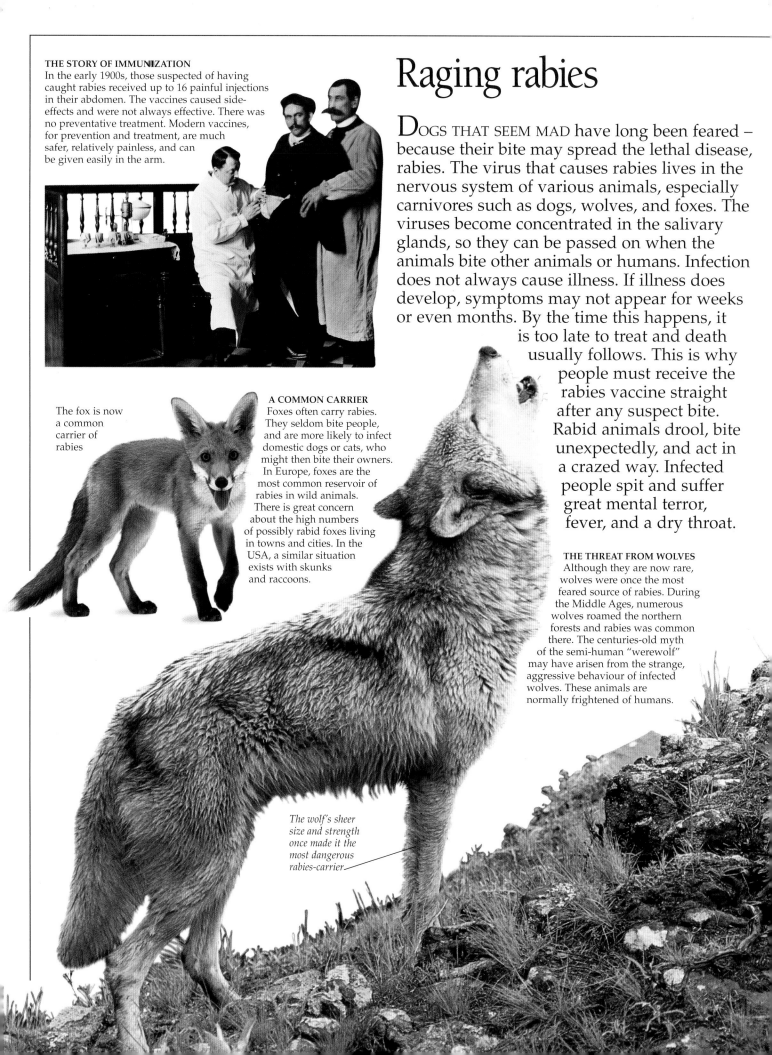

DOGS THAT SEEM MAD have long been feared – because their bite may spread the lethal disease, rabies. The virus that causes rabies lives in the nervous system of various animals, especially carnivores such as dogs, wolves, and foxes. The viruses become concentrated in the salivary glands, so they can be passed on when the animals bite other animals or humans. Infection does not always cause illness. If illness does develop, symptoms may not appear for weeks or even months. By the time this happens, it is too late to treat and death usually follows. This is why people must receive the rabies vaccine straight after any suspect bite. Rabid animals drool, bite unexpectedly, and act in a crazed way. Infected people spit and suffer great mental terror, fever, and a dry throat.

The fox is now a common carrier of rabies

A COMMON CARRIER
Foxes often carry rabies. They seldom bite people, and are more likely to infect domestic dogs or cats, who might then bite their owners. In Europe, foxes are the most common reservoir of rabies in wild animals. There is great concern about the high numbers of possibly rabid foxes living in towns and cities. In the USA, a similar situation exists with skunks and raccoons.

THE THREAT FROM WOLVES
Although they are now rare, wolves were once the most feared source of rabies. During the Middle Ages, numerous wolves roamed the northern forests and rabies was common there. The centuries-old myth of the semi-human "werewolf" may have arisen from the strange, aggressive behaviour of infected wolves. These animals are normally frightened of humans.

The wolf's sheer size and strength once made it the most dangerous rabies-carrier

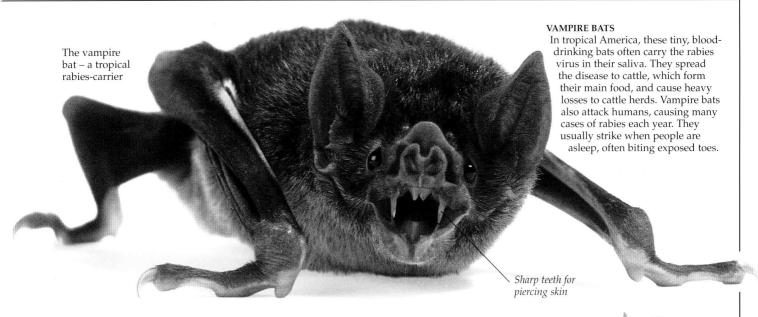

The vampire bat – a tropical rabies-carrier

VAMPIRE BATS
In tropical America, these tiny, blood-drinking bats often carry the rabies virus in their saliva. They spread the disease to cattle, which form their main food, and cause heavy losses to cattle herds. Vampire bats also attack humans, causing many cases of rabies each year. They usually strike when people are asleep, often biting exposed toes.

Sharp teeth for piercing skin

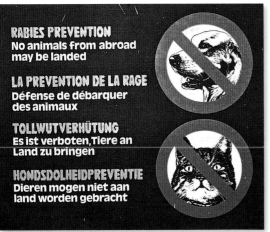

RABIES PREVENTION
No animals from abroad may be landed

LA PREVENTION DE LA RAGE
Défense de débarquer des animaux

TOLLWUTVERHÜTUNG
Es ist verboten, Tiere an Land zu bringen

HONDSDOLHEIDPREVENTIE
Dieren mogen niet aan land worden gebracht

KEEPING RABIES OUT
Notices like this appear at ports, airports, and borders. They explain which animals cannot be brought into a country because they may be infected with – and spread – diseases such as rabies. Those that are let in may be held in quarantine (secure pens) for a time to see if any disease develops. This is most effective on islands, where there is less chance of infected wild animals wandering into the country. Now that better vaccines exist, quarantine may no longer be so important.

NATURAL RABIES REMEDY
The ancient Greeks tried to treat rabies with extracts from the aptly named dog rose plant. Other historical treatments included burning out tissue around the bite, which may have prevented infection from developing. One doctor even suggested filling a wound with gunpowder and setting it alight!

Dog Rose
(*Rosa canina*)

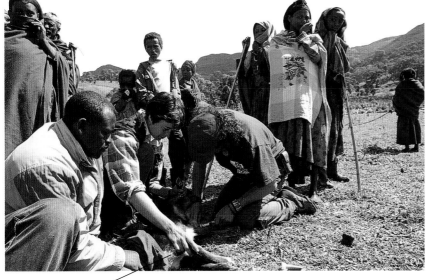

VACCINATING DOGS
This veterinary team is travelling around an infected part of Ethiopia, vaccinating every dog to reduce the risk to humans. Because dogs mix so closely with people, they can be a serious threat. New, effective vaccines have been developed that stop the disease from spreading between dogs. In some countries, vaccinated animals are given "passports" to show that they are protected from rabies.

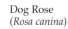

Vets who vaccinate potentially rabid dogs have to be vaccinated against rabies themselves, in case the dogs are already rabid

LATEST RABIES RESEARCH
One of the latest developments in the fight against rabies is a vaccine for animals that can be given by mouth. This vaccine can be incorporated into food pellets. The pellets are then dropped by aeroplanes over areas where rabies affects foxes. Although a vaccination for rabies has existed since Louis Pasteur developed one in the late 1800s, constant research is still being carried out into better ways to protect both people and animals from the disease.

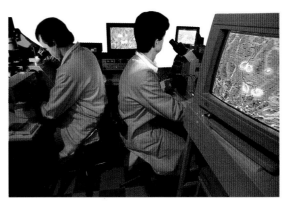

Coughs and colds

LOTS OF DIFFERENT ORGANISMS can cause coughs and colds, even though the symptoms may feel much the same. What all these conditions have in common is that they are infections of the upper respiratory tract – that is, they affect the breathing passages above the lungs. Viruses are usually responsible – over 100 different types cause coughs and colds – and these cannot be destroyed by antibiotics. Although we quickly develop natural immunity after a viral infection, we will not be immune to the next type of virus we encounter. Some bacteria are culprits, such as *Staphylococcus*, and these will respond to drugs if symptoms become too uncomfortable. Young children may get several different infections every year, especially once they come into contact with other children at school.

NATURAL REMEDIES
Eucalyptus is one of the aromatic plants that can soothe cold symptoms. It is usually the natural oils extracted from these plants that are used in remedies. They may be included in soothing, anti-inflammatory throat pastilles or inhaled to help clear passages blocked by swelling and mucus.

An adenovirus – one of the viruses that cause the common cold

SYMPTOMS AND EFFECTS
In the event of a cold, it is usually the head and throat that suffer most. Coughs and colds usually start with a virus attack. This produces fever and inflammation of the lining of the nose and of air filled spaces called sinuses. The linings produce lots of mucus as a result, making the nose run and causing uncomfortable blockage of the sinuses. Bacteria may also attack inflamed areas, leading to painful sinuses, coughing, and sore throats.

Large protruding proteins (antigens) on surface trigger the immune system

Spherical shape

Sinuses are blocked and swollen and may become infected

Nose and nasal passages fill with mucus and nose starts running

Throat, or pharynx, may become infected with Streptococcus *bacteria*

NON-NATURAL CURES
Drug treatments bought over the counter or prescribed by doctors cost billions of pounds each year. Most of these are intended to ease or disguise symptoms. They can reduce inflammation, ease aches and pains, and dry up runny noses. They rarely tackle the root of the problem. The body will usually cure itself of viral infections after just a few days. However, bacteria may step in at this point, preying on already damaged tissues and sometimes making medical treatment necessary.

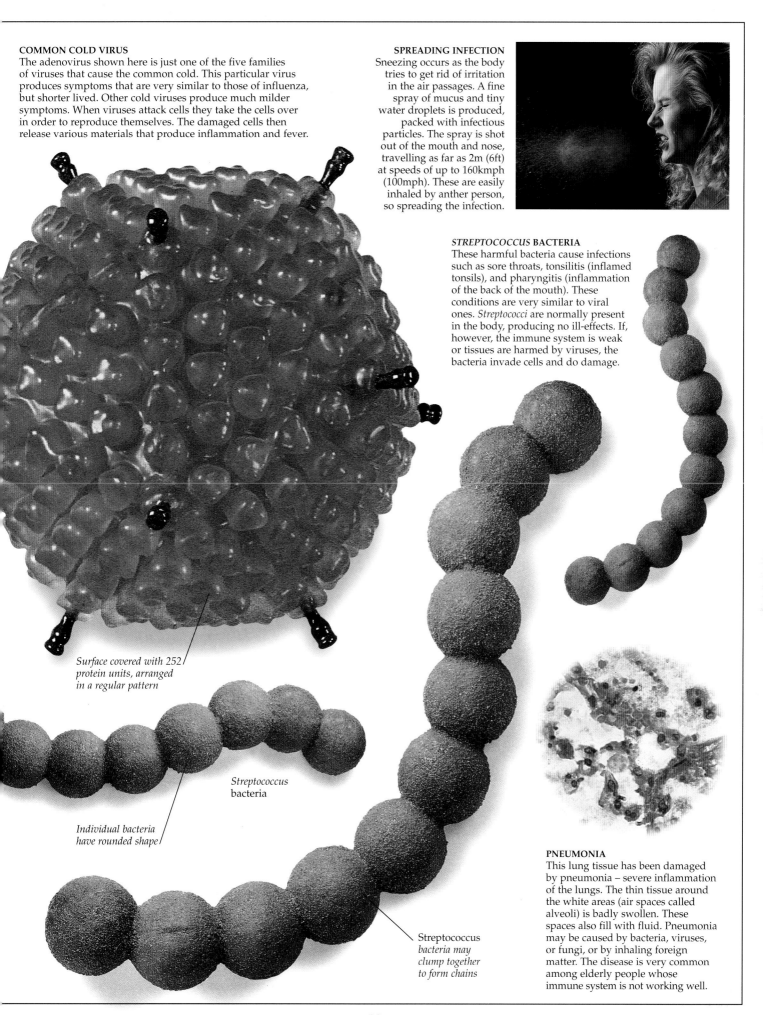

COMMON COLD VIRUS
The adenovirus shown here is just one of the five families of viruses that cause the common cold. This particular virus produces symptoms that are very similar to those of influenza, but shorter lived. Other cold viruses produce much milder symptoms. When viruses attack cells they take the cells over in order to reproduce themselves. The damaged cells then release various materials that produce inflammation and fever.

SPREADING INFECTION
Sneezing occurs as the body tries to get rid of irritation in the air passages. A fine spray of mucus and tiny water droplets is produced, packed with infectious particles. The spray is shot out of the mouth and nose, travelling as far as 2m (6ft) at speeds of up to 160kmph (100mph). These are easily inhaled by anther person, so spreading the infection.

***STREPTOCOCCUS* BACTERIA**
These harmful bacteria cause infections such as sore throats, tonsilitis (inflamed tonsils), and pharyngitis (inflammation of the back of the mouth). These conditions are very similar to viral ones. *Streptococci* are normally present in the body, producing no ill-effects. If, however, the immune system is weak or tissues are harmed by viruses, the bacteria invade cells and do damage.

Surface covered with 252 protein units, arranged in a regular pattern

Streptococcus bacteria

Individual bacteria have rounded shape

Streptococcus bacteria may clump together to form chains

PNEUMONIA
This lung tissue has been damaged by pneumonia – severe inflammation of the lungs. The thin tissue around the white areas (air spaces called alveoli) is badly swollen. These spaces also fill with fluid. Pneumonia may be caused by bacteria, viruses, or fungi, or by inhaling foreign matter. The disease is very common among elderly people whose immune system is not working well.

Influenza

Many PEOPLE CLAIM TO HAVE influenza, or flu, when all they actually have is a bad cold. Like many colds, flu is a viral illness, but it is more severe and longer lasting. Symptoms are fever, aching muscles, and a cough. Sufferers usually feel tired and weak for a while after the symptoms have disappeared. As with all viral diseases, any medicines will only ease the symptoms, and cannot wipe out the cause. Flu tends to break out in epidemics and there have been some serious ones in the past. Most people can cope with flu, but the very young, the elderly, and those with respiratory problems can become very ill. Many vulnerable people are encouraged to have a flu vaccination each year.

FLU FUMIGATOR
Around 1900, people used fumigators like this to try to kill flu-causing microbes in the air. Various substances were put inside and heated to produce strong fumes. People at this time did not understand the cause of flu and other lung infections and these devices were completely ineffective.

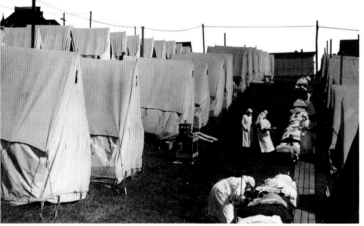

THE FLU PANDEMIC OF 1918–1920
Taken in 1918, this picture shows an army isolation hospital in Maine, USA, where troops are being treated for flu. The flu pandemic of 1918–1920 was the worst outbreak that anyone at the time could recall. It swept the whole world and affected many troops serving in World War I (1914–1918). The war killed 15 million people, while the flu killed at least 20 million.

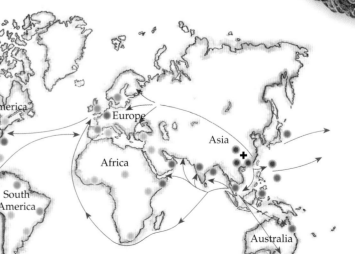

Where it began, in February 1957 ✚

Where flu had spread after 0–2 months ●

Where flu had spread after 3–4 months ●

Where flu had spread after 5–6 months ●

Where flu had spread after 7–8 months ●

North America

Europe

Asia

Africa

South America

Australia

THE FLU PANDEMIC OF 1957–1958
The spread of this pandemic followed a pattern that is common for flu epidemics. It first appeared in Southeast Asia and travelled to cities such as Hong Kong and Singapore. From these major ports it was carried farther afield on ships and aircraft and in a few months was all over the globe. Many epidemics start in Southeast Asia because they often begin life in animals such as ducks, chickens, and pigs. Flu viruses switch easily from animals to humans, and these animals live in close association with people in this part of the world.

How flu swept the world in 1957

THE FLU VIRUS

Flu is caused by strains of myxovirus. These are grouped as types A, B, and C, with Type A being the most common cause. Immunity from one strain does not protect against another. Flu viruses can change form very rapidly, into strains for which people have no immunity. Every 30 years or so a strain appears that no one is immune to, and a pandemic occurs.

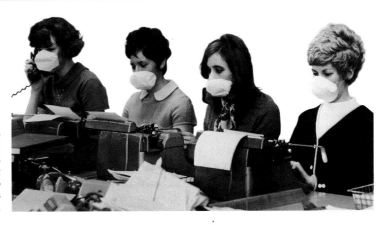

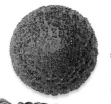

STOPPING THE SPREAD

These masked office workers were photographed during a flu epidemic of the 1960s. As the virus is spread by water droplets coughed up or sneezed out by infected people, masks were once handed out to prevent infection. Unfortunately, this is ineffective as the tiny viruses can passes through any type of filter.

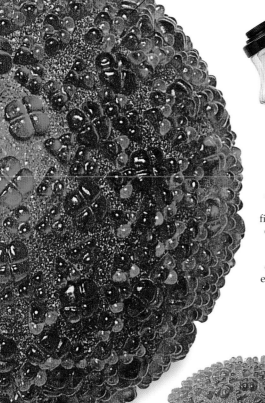

Round shape

ANTI-FLU MOUTHPIECES

This sanitary mouthpiece was designed to keep the mouth away from a potentially infected telephone handset. It was once thought that diseases such as flu could be caught by contact with items that had been used by an infected person. In practice, it is unlikely that the infection could be caught in this way.

The scientists used ground-penetrating radar to locate victims' coffins

FROZEN EVIDENCE

In 1998, scientists dug up the bodies of Norwegian flu victims from the 1918 pandemic. The bodies were well preserved in Norway's frozen climate and contained remains of the virus. These findings have been studied by experts as part of an ongoing effort to stop this virus from striking again. The 1918 outbreak has always puzzled experts because it vanished as mysteriously as it appeared.

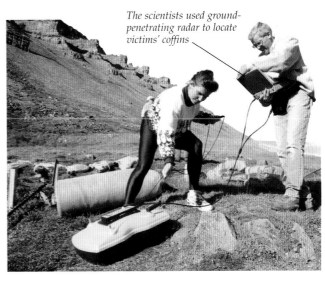

Surface covered with antigens that the immune system may, or may not, recognize

Protein coat surrounds each virus

Generalized model of a myxovirus

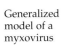

ASIAN FLU VIRUSES

This is a group of the type of virus that has caused "Hong Kong Flu", just one of the forms of flu that emerges from Asia every few years. Asian flu viruses are all similar in appearance. A core of genetic material is surrounded by a spiky coat of protein. This coat helps the virus to stick to cells in the lungs – flu viruses principally attack the lungs and the passages of the respiratory system.

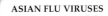

35

Attacking the brain

THE DELICATE BRAIN IS GENERALLY well protected against infection. A finely balanced exchange system exists in the human brain, which prevents most harmful intruders from entering brain tissue via the blood vessels that run through it. However, some diseases do get through and may cause severe brain damage, even death. Meningitis, caused either by a virus or a bacterium, is one of the most common diseases affecting the brain. Even normally mild childhood diseases such as measles occasionally enter the brain and cause harm, sometimes years after the original infection. Today, the use of antibiotics usually stops a disease from getting as far as causing brain-damage.

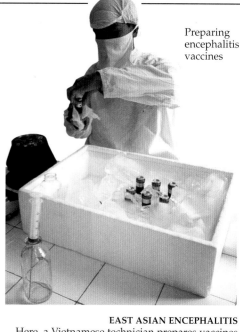

Preparing encephalitis vaccines

EAST ASIAN ENCEPHALITIS
Here, a Vietnamese technician prepares vaccines against Japanese encephalitis B. This serious viral disease can cause fever, drowsiness, and possible brain damage. Mosquitoes pick the virus up from infected birds and pigs and then pass it to humans by biting. It causes major epidemics in eastern Asia, where virus-carrying mosquitoes thrive around the rice fields. Other forms of encephalitis occur elsewhere and most are caused by viruses.

THE CENTRAL NERVOUS SYSTEM
The long spinal cord, and the brain positioned at the top of it, make up the central nervous system, or CNS. A vast network of interconnecting nerves within this system controls the functioning of our whole body. Infections that get into the nervous system are particularly dangerous because they prevent the rest of the body from working properly.

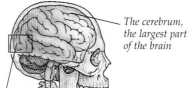

The cerebrum, the largest part of the brain

Area that is shown enlarged on right

THE BRAIN AND THE MENINGES
Three membranes, the meninges, protect the brain and spinal cord. The outer layer (dura mater) is very tough and contains many blood vessels. The middle layer (arachnoid) is net-like and rubbery, while the inner layer (pia mater) is thin and delicate. Meningitis is named after these membranes. In this, and certain other brain diseases, the infected membranes swell and press painfully against the skull.

Dura mater *Arachnoid* *Pia Mater* *Skull*

Cerebrum

Large blood vessel

Bone of skull *Area that contains cushioning cerebrospinal fluid and blood vessels*

BACTERIAL MENINGITIS
Neisseria meningitidis is one of the bacteria that cause meningitis. Bacterial forms of the disease can be very serious, producing fever, a stiff neck, rash, headache, and vomiting, even death. If caught early, this can be treated with antibiotics. Viral meningitis is usually much milder and flu-like.

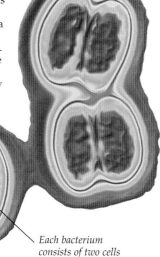

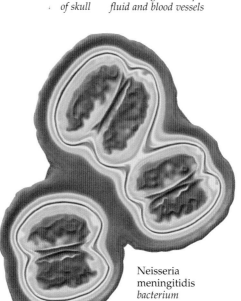

Each bacterium consists of two cells in a round capsule

Neisseria meningitidis bacterium

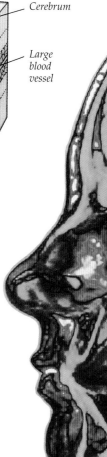

ENCEPHALITIS ON FILM

Awakenings depicts the results of a mysterious form of encephalitis that swept the world in the 1920s. It killed some people, while others fell into a coma or a zombie-like state. A drug called levodopa brought some patients "back to life", but only for a short while. The problem vanished as mysteriously as it arrived. We still do not know the cause and, as far as is known, this illness has never recurred.

From the 1990 US film, *Awakenings*, with Robert DeNiro (left) and Robin Williams (right)

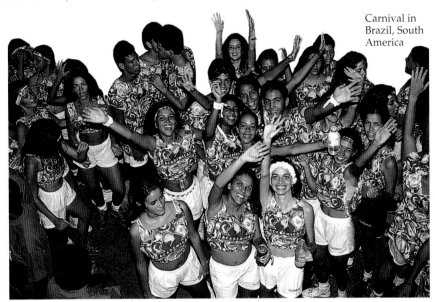

Carnival in Brazil, South America

HAVING FUN SAFELY

Big international carnivals can provide a breeding ground for dangerous microbes. When people go home, they take diseases with them. In 1974, a huge meningitis epidemic struck Brazil. There were great fears that the annual Rio carnival would speed its spread. A vast vaccination programme was mounted – three million people were vaccinated within five days – and this brought the epidemic to a halt.

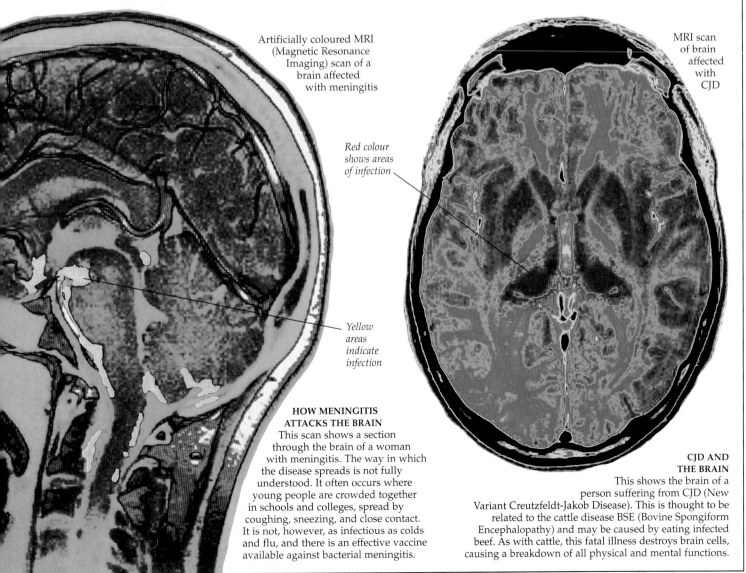

Artificially coloured MRI (Magnetic Resonance Imaging) scan of a brain affected with meningitis

MRI scan of brain affected with CJD

Red colour shows areas of infection

Yellow areas indicate infection

HOW MENINGITIS ATTACKS THE BRAIN

This scan shows a section through the brain of a woman with meningitis. The way in which the disease spreads is not fully understood. It often occurs where young people are crowded together in schools and colleges, spread by coughing, sneezing, and close contact. It is not, however, as infectious as colds and flu, and there is an effective vaccine available against bacterial meningitis.

CJD AND THE BRAIN

This shows the brain of a person suffering from CJD (New Variant Creutzfeldt-Jakob Disease). This is thought to be related to the cattle disease BSE (Bovine Spongiform Encephalopathy) and may be caused by eating infected beef. As with cattle, this fatal illness destroys brain cells, causing a breakdown of all physical and mental functions.

Childhood diseases

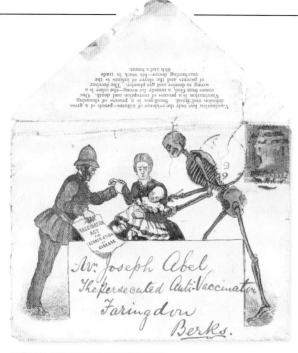

THERE IS A PARTICULAR GROUP OF DISEASES that are common in children – including chickenpox, mumps, and measles. Some of these are caused by bacteria, others by viruses. After children have successfully recovered from one of these illnesses, they usually have life-long immunity from it. Most childhood diseases are highly infectious and are spread by contact – often when children play together. Many such infections are easily prevented by means of routine vaccinations. If they do cause illness, it is seldom serious or may be treated with antibiotics. It is not that long ago – the 1930s – that certain infections killed children, even in medically advanced countries. These infections included diphtheria, scarlet fever, and whooping cough. They can still be dangerous in poorer countries, so health agencies do what they can to organize widescale vaccination programmes in vulnerable areas.

ANTI-VACCINATION CAMPAIGNS
This envelope was part of an 1899 anti-vaccination campaign. The flap states that vaccination is a "fraud". There have always been people who have opposed vaccinations, because some children have become ill as a result of receiving them. However, there is much less chance of this today, and a far greater risk of death because people have not been vaccinated.

DIPHTHERIA VACCINE
A modern diphtheria vaccine. Diphtheria is just one of the old killer diseases that can now be routinely prevented by widescale vaccination of children.

This vaccine combats both diptheria and tetanus

CHILD VACCINATION
These children are queuing up at school to be vaccinated against TB in the 1950s. Widescale vaccination programmes for many common childhood diseases got off the ground between the 1930s and the 1960s. Once a majority of people carry the antibodies to a disease, that disease tends to die out completely for a long time, apart from isolated cases.

Vaccines are injected into an area of muscle. The top of the arm is usually the most accessible place to give a vaccination

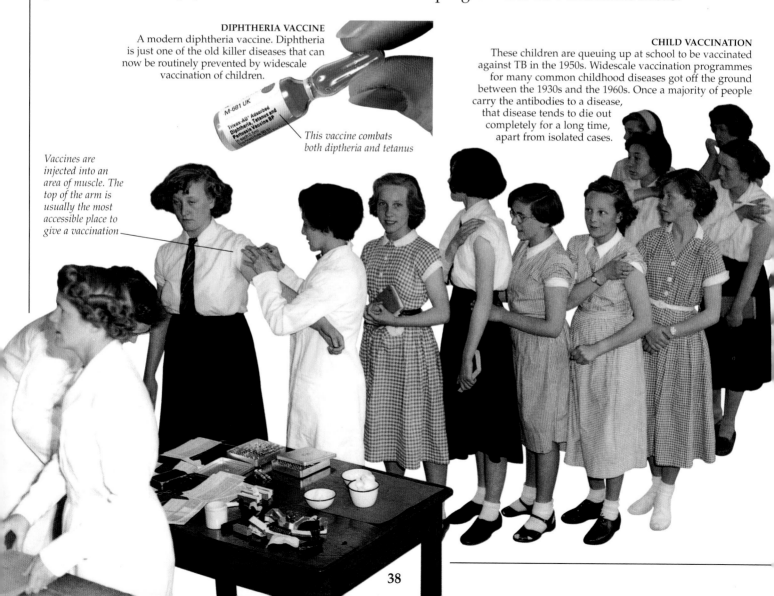

MEASLES VIRUS

The virus that causes measles is closely related to the viruses causing distemper in dogs and rinderpest in African cattle. Once very common, measles is now rare in the world's richer countries, due to widespread vaccination. However, it does still kill in poorer countries. Because measles only affects humans, there is no animal reservoir of the virus. This means that there is a real possibility that the disease could be wiped out by global vaccination programmes.

Virus from the *Morbillivirus* group

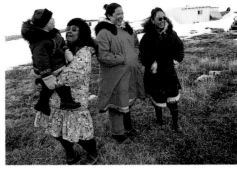

ISOLATED COMMUNITIES

These are Inuit people from Alaska, in the far north-west of the USA. In the past, Inuit communities have been wiped out by diseases such as measles. This is because remote peoples who have never been affected before have no immunity. Vaccination campaigns have done much to help this situation.

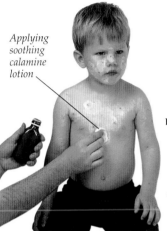

Applying soothing calamine lotion

DEALING WITH SYMPTOMS

Rashes are common with childhood infections such as rubella and chickenpox. These rashes are non-threatening but may be very itchy. The irritation can be reduced by dabbing on a soothing preparation. Calamine lotion is a traditional remedy that has been used for many years.

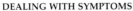

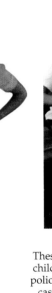

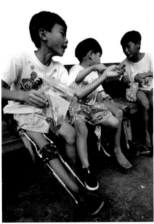

POLIOMYELITIS (POLIO)

These partially paralyzed Vietnamese children were not immunized against polio. They are suffering from a severe case of this viral disease, which has affected their nervous system. The polio vaccine is dropped onto the tongue or taken on a lump of sugar.

WHOOPING COUGH BACTERIUM

The *Bordetella pertussis* bacterium causes a serious infection of the air passages. Affecting mainly babies and young children, it makes breathing difficult and produces a cough with a strange "whooping" sound. Vaccination normally occurs in a child's first year.

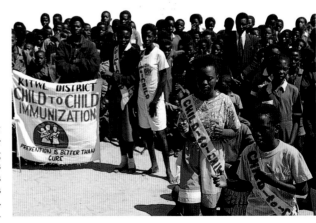

GLOBAL IMMUNIZATION

Here, ordinary people in Zambia, southern Africa, show their support for a child immunization (vaccination) programme taking place in their area. Disease control throughout the world means painstakingly checking, treating, and vaccinating people. As diseases come under control in certain regions, medical teams go out into ever more remote areas where the illness persists, vaccinating people and following up any reports of infection.

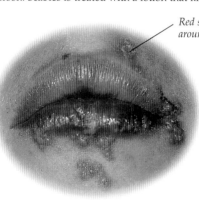

A scabies mite burrows through skin

Human hair

Skin cells

The scabies mite, Sarcoptes scabiei

Minor plagues

WE ARE USUALLY CONCERNED about disease-causing microbes living inside us. However, there are all kinds of organisms that sometimes find their way onto the surface of our bodies, too. These parasitic microbes create a range of health problems that are mostly mild but often very irritating. Nearly all of these creatures are spread by touch. This means that they often affect children, who pick up microbes easily as they play together. At one time, nearly everyone would have carried these parasites. We no longer tolerate such obvious intruders, and modern hygiene methods usually keep them under control. This is important because serious diseases like typhus have been spread by lice, and the plague by flea bites.

HOW SCABIES GETS UNDER THE SKIN
This model shows how the skin disease scabies arises. Scabies is caused by a tiny mite, about 0.5mm (⅕₀in) long. It burrows through the skin, just under the surface, and lays eggs there. The mite produces tiny, winding tunnels, which may cause grey swellings on the skin's surface. These tunnels often become infected, and this produces intense itching. Scratching affected areas releases the eggs, which may then be picked up by another person. Scabies is treated with a lotion that kills the mites.

Red sores on and around mouth

COLD SORES
Unsightly, painful sores sometimes appear on and around the mouth. These are usually caused by the herpes simplex Type 1 virus, which is passed from one person to another by close contact. Once inside the body, the virus stays there. The immune system can normally cope with it, but sores break out if a person is run down and so has a weak immune system.

VERRUCAS
Verrucas are warts – common skin-growths – that are found on the sole of the foot. Unlike ordinary warts, they grow inwards, under the pressure of walking about. They can become very painful. Verrucas are caused by the wart virus. This likes warm, damp conditions and is often found in swimming pools and gym changing rooms.

Hard growth known as a verruca

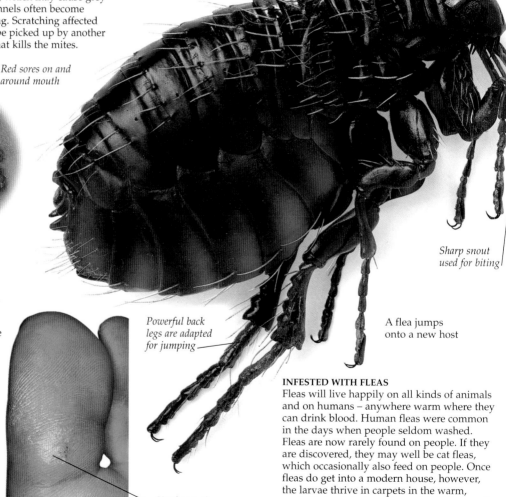

Sharp snout used for biting

Powerful back legs are adapted for jumping

A flea jumps onto a new host

INFESTED WITH FLEAS
Fleas will live happily on all kinds of animals and on humans – anywhere warm where they can drink blood. Human fleas were common in the days when people seldom washed. Fleas are now rarely found on people. If they are discovered, they may well be cat fleas, which occasionally also feed on people. Once fleas do get into a modern house, however, the larvae thrive in carpets in the warm, centrally heated atmosphere. Adult fleas make tiny wounds when they bite. These often itch, and scratching them can cause skin infections.

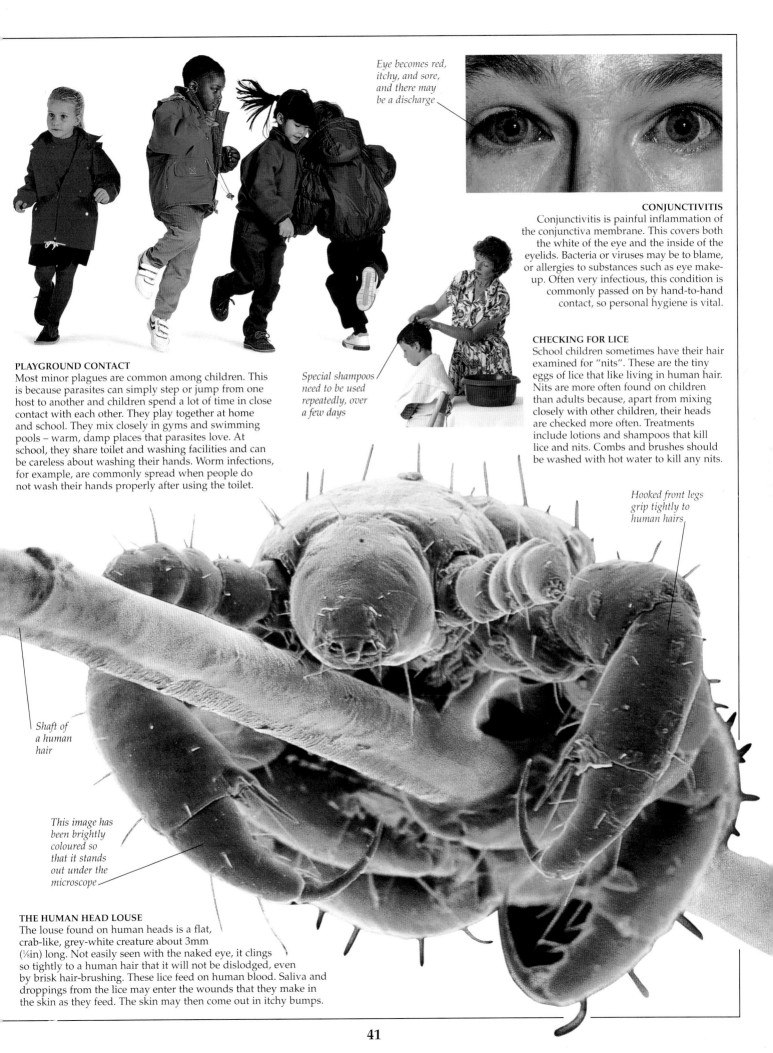

Eye becomes red, itchy, and sore, and there may be a discharge

CONJUNCTIVITIS

Conjunctivitis is painful inflammation of the conjunctiva membrane. This covers both the white of the eye and the inside of the eyelids. Bacteria or viruses may be to blame, or allergies to substances such as eye make-up. Often very infectious, this condition is commonly passed on by hand-to-hand contact, so personal hygiene is vital.

CHECKING FOR LICE

School children sometimes have their hair examined for "nits". These are the tiny eggs of lice that like living in human hair. Nits are more often found on children than adults because, apart from mixing closely with other children, their heads are checked more often. Treatments include lotions and shampoos that kill lice and nits. Combs and brushes should be washed with hot water to kill any nits.

Special shampoos need to be used repeatedly, over a few days

PLAYGROUND CONTACT

Most minor plagues are common among children. This is because parasites can simply step or jump from one host to another and children spend a lot of time in close contact with each other. They play together at home and school. They mix closely in gyms and swimming pools – warm, damp places that parasites love. At school, they share toilet and washing facilities and can be careless about washing their hands. Worm infections, for example, are commonly spread when people do not wash their hands properly after using the toilet.

Hooked front legs grip tightly to human hairs

Shaft of a human hair

This image has been brightly coloured so that it stands out under the microscope

THE HUMAN HEAD LOUSE

The louse found on human heads is a flat, crab-like, grey-white creature about 3mm (⅛in) long. Not easily seen with the naked eye, it clings so tightly to a human hair that it will not be dislodged, even by brisk hair-brushing. These lice feed on human blood. Saliva and droppings from the lice may enter the wounds that they make in the skin as they feed. The skin may then come out in itchy bumps.

Deadly bugs

Undulating membrane

MANY OF THE DEADLIEST diseases are spread by the bites of mosquitoes, ticks, lice, and flies. They carry infectious microbes that are injected into humans when they bite. Most of these diseases also affect animals, which act as reservoirs of infection, making the disease difficult to stamp out. African sleeping sickness, or trypanosomiasis, is a typical disease of this type. There are several forms of sleeping sickness, but it mostly affects cattle and game animals in tropical Africa. When the tsetse fly feeds on an infected animal's blood, then bites a human, the tiny *Trypanosoma* parasite is injected into the bloodstream and begins to multiply. This causes illness and possibly inflammation of the brain. The sufferer becomes sleepy and falls into a coma. This disease can be successfully treated with drugs. To reduce the chance of being bitten, people must use insecticide, cover up, and avoid areas where groups of this day-feeding fly are gathering.

These parasites swim by making wave-like movements

DR WALTER REED
In the early 1900s, this American doctor helped to prove that yellow fever was spread by mosquito bites. Reed was serving on a special commission, set up by the US government to find the cause of yellow fever because so many troops had died from the disease. Reed's discovery also made it possible to complete the Panama Canal, in 1914. Progress on this had been halted by yellow fever and malaria among the workers. When scrub along the canal was cleared, and pools where mosquitoes bred were drained, illness rates fell dramatically.

BODY LICE AND TYPHUS
Typhus is mostly spread by lice that cling to human body hair, although some forms are spread by fleas. The lice pass on a tiny *Rickettsia* organism when they bite. Typhus often occurs in unhygienic places where people are crowded together, so epidemics have often broken out in poor cities and during wars. Symptoms of this serious disease include fever and internal bleeding. Use of insecticides and antibiotics have reduced its incidence greatly over the years.

Tube called proboscis, through which blood is sucked

Abdomen swollen with blood that the fly has sucked up

Visible to the naked eye, the louse Pediculus humanus is one of the carriers that spreads typhus

TSETSE FLY AND SLEEPING SICKNESS
Tsetse flies spread sleeping sickness via their bite. This fly is a relative of the ordinary house fly. It carries the *Trypanosoma* parasite in its salivary glands for up to 96 days. During this time, it can infect everyone it bites. Tsetse flies live in damp areas along the banks of rivers and lakes. They sometimes swarm in such numbers that an area becomes uninhabitable. Insecticides are widely used to control them.

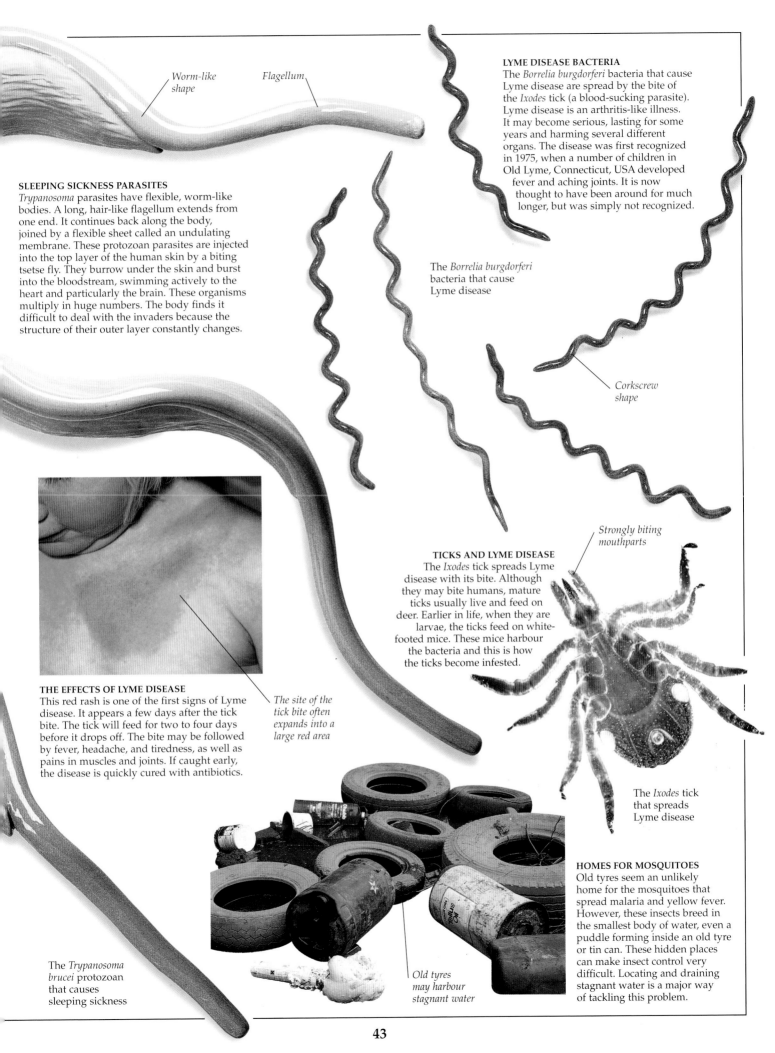

SLEEPING SICKNESS PARASITES

Trypanosoma parasites have flexible, worm-like bodies. A long, hair-like flagellum extends from one end. It continues back along the body, joined by a flexible sheet called an undulating membrane. These protozoan parasites are injected into the top layer of the human skin by a biting tsetse fly. They burrow under the skin and burst into the bloodstream, swimming actively to the heart and particularly the brain. These organisms multiply in huge numbers. The body finds it difficult to deal with the invaders because the structure of their outer layer constantly changes.

Worm-like shape

Flagellum

LYME DISEASE BACTERIA

The *Borrelia burgdorferi* bacteria that cause Lyme disease are spread by the bite of the *Ixodes* tick (a blood-sucking parasite). Lyme disease is an arthritis-like illness. It may become serious, lasting for some years and harming several different organs. The disease was first recognized in 1975, when a number of children in Old Lyme, Connecticut, USA developed fever and aching joints. It is now thought to have been around for much longer, but was simply not recognized.

The *Borrelia burgdorferi* bacteria that cause Lyme disease

Corkscrew shape

Strongly biting mouthparts

TICKS AND LYME DISEASE

The *Ixodes* tick spreads Lyme disease with its bite. Although they may bite humans, mature ticks usually live and feed on deer. Earlier in life, when they are larvae, the ticks feed on white-footed mice. These mice harbour the bacteria and this is how the ticks become infested.

THE EFFECTS OF LYME DISEASE

This red rash is one of the first signs of Lyme disease. It appears a few days after the tick bite. The tick will feed for two to four days before it drops off. The bite may be followed by fever, headache, and tiredness, as well as pains in muscles and joints. If caught early, the disease is quickly cured with antibiotics.

The site of the tick bite often expands into a large red area

The *Ixodes* tick that spreads Lyme disease

HOMES FOR MOSQUITOES

Old tyres seem an unlikely home for the mosquitoes that spread malaria and yellow fever. However, these insects breed in the smallest body of water, even a puddle forming inside an old tyre or tin can. These hidden places can make insect control very difficult. Locating and draining stagnant water is a major way of tackling this problem.

The *Trypanosoma brucei* protozoan that causes sleeping sickness

Old tyres may harbour stagnant water

Dealing with worms

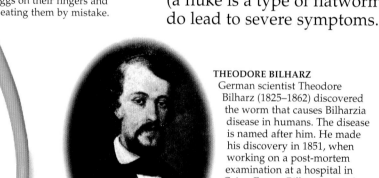

MOST ORGANISMS THAT PRODUCE DISEASE are single-celled and microscopically small. Disease-causing worms, however, are multi-celled creatures that can grow to lengths of 12m (40ft). They are parasites – surviving by living in the bodies of certain animals and people – and some are the largest known agents of human disease. Worms found inside people are either flatworms or roundworms. Humans pick up parasitic worm eggs, larvae, or mature worms from infected food, water, or soil. Most worms have adapted to living inside humans without causing too much damage and people may have them for many years without knowing. Infestations usually produce general ill-health rather than serious disease, but some, such as the Bilharzia fluke (a fluke is a type of flatworm), do lead to severe symptoms.

Slim, round shape

COMMON ROUNDWORM
These worms are around the size of a pencil. They live in human intestines, gaining nourishment from the food we eat. Common roundworms usually cause significant symptoms only if they are present in large numbers. Children often become infected when they touch dog or cat faeces (or soil tainted with faeces), picking up worm eggs on their fingers and eating them by mistake.

Common ascarid roundworm

Very simple body consists basically of a long digestive tube with a head at one end and an anus at the other

THEODORE BILHARZ
German scientist Theodore Bilharz (1825–1862) discovered the worm that causes Bilharzia disease in humans. The disease is named after him. He made his discovery in 1851, when working on a post-mortem examination at a hospital in Cairo, Egypt. Bilharz noticed numerous white worms in a major blood vessel supplying the liver "which I immediately recognized as something new."

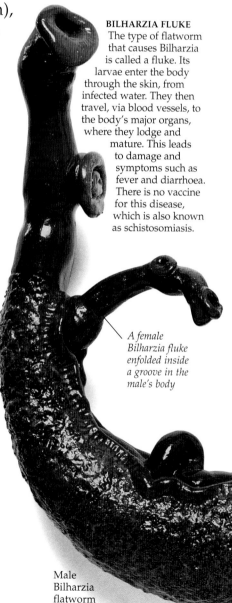

BILHARZIA FLUKE
The type of flatworm that causes Bilharzia is called a fluke. Its larvae enter the body through the skin, from infected water. They then travel, via blood vessels, to the body's major organs, where they lodge and mature. This leads to damage and symptoms such as fever and diarrhoea. There is no vaccine for this disease, which is also known as schistosomiasis.

A female Bilharzia fluke enfolded inside a groove in the male's body

Male Bilharzia flatworm

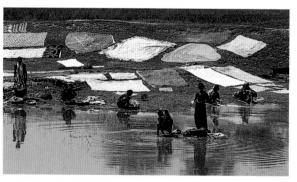

RISK FROM WATER
Many diseases are spread via water – especially where people swim, wash, and clean clothes in the same body of water. Bilharzia larvae, for example, infect people who swim in infested rivers and lakes. These people may deposit worm eggs in the water in their faeces or urine. The eggs develop into larvae, which burrow into water snails and multiply there. They then emerge and swim off to find new human hosts.

DAMS AND DISEASE
Dams are vital all over the world for hydroelectric power and for irrigating the land. Unfortunately, the water snails that help to spread Bilharzia often thrive in the still waters held back by large dams, and it seems that incidence of the disease is rising as more dams and water projects are constructed. Bilharzia is a major problem in tropical regions and attempts have been made to control it by destroying the snails.

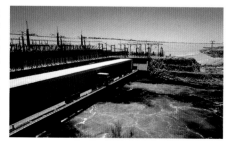

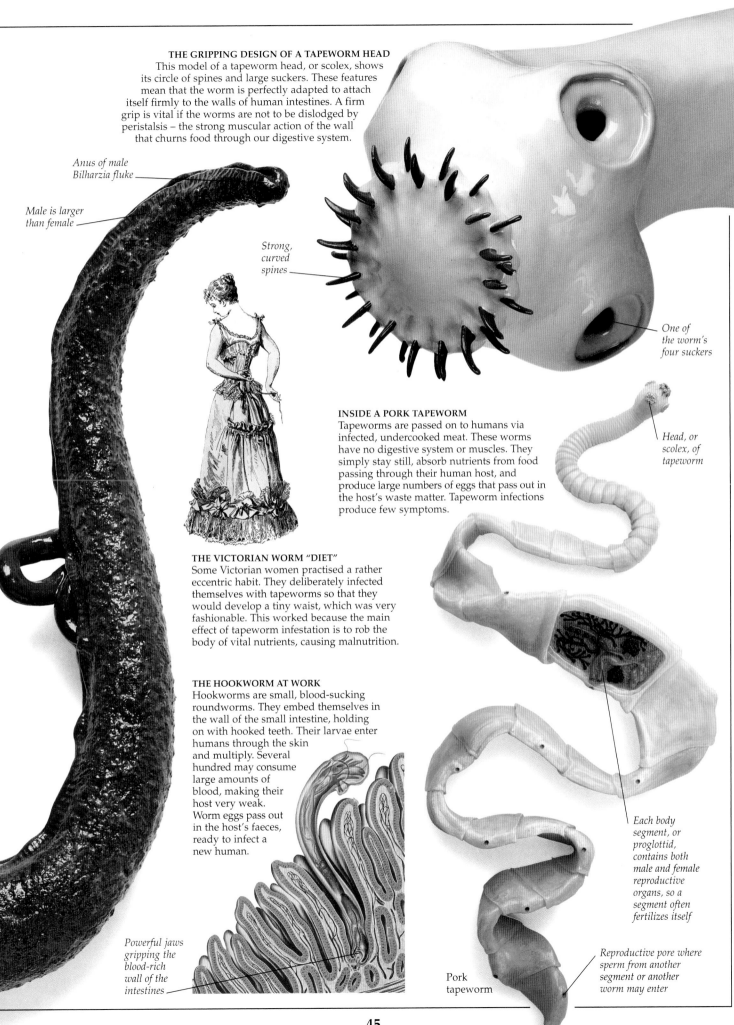

THE GRIPPING DESIGN OF A TAPEWORM HEAD
This model of a tapeworm head, or scolex, shows its circle of spines and large suckers. These features mean that the worm is perfectly adapted to attach itself firmly to the walls of human intestines. A firm grip is vital if the worms are not to be dislodged by peristalsis – the strong muscular action of the wall that churns food through our digestive system.

Anus of male Bilharzia fluke

Male is larger than female

Strong, curved spines

One of the worm's four suckers

INSIDE A PORK TAPEWORM
Tapeworms are passed on to humans via infected, undercooked meat. These worms have no digestive system or muscles. They simply stay still, absorb nutrients from food passing through their human host, and produce large numbers of eggs that pass out in the host's waste matter. Tapeworm infections produce few symptoms.

Head, or scolex, of tapeworm

THE VICTORIAN WORM "DIET"
Some Victorian women practised a rather eccentric habit. They deliberately infected themselves with tapeworms so that they would develop a tiny waist, which was very fashionable. This worked because the main effect of tapeworm infestation is to rob the body of vital nutrients, causing malnutrition.

THE HOOKWORM AT WORK
Hookworms are small, blood-sucking roundworms. They embed themselves in the wall of the small intestine, holding on with hooked teeth. Their larvae enter humans through the skin and multiply. Several hundred may consume large amounts of blood, making their host very weak. Worm eggs pass out in the host's faeces, ready to infect a new human.

Each body segment, or proglottid, contains both male and female reproductive organs, so a segment often fertilizes itself

Reproductive pore where sperm from another segment or another worm may enter

Powerful jaws gripping the blood-rich wall of the intestines

Pork tapeworm

Malaria

THIS DISEASE IS SPREAD BY the bite of female *Anopheles* mosquitoes, in warm, humid parts of the world. Their bite passes on disease-causing parasites living inside the mosquito. The parasite may stay dormant in a person's liver for months or even years before symptoms appear. People do develop some immunity to malaria, but only to a particular strain. There are several forms of malaria, all causing fever, shivering, and weakness. In some, the symptoms vanish quickly, then reappear several weeks later. These forms may persist for many years. Other, more serious, types can kill if they are not treated quickly – this is a curable illness if it is caught early enough. Worldwide, 500 million cases of the disease appear each year, making malaria a major health issue. Problems arise when the parasites become resistant to drugs. This is why prevention is so vital. Educating people to use anti-malarial drugs, nets, and insect-repellent has been shown to make all the difference.

How malaria-causing parasites pass from red cells to the bloodstream

PASSING ON THE PARASITE
The female *Anopheles* mosquito lands on human skin and sucks up blood through needle-shaped mouthparts. The mosquito injects saliva into the wound as it sucks. In the saliva are malarial parasites, which pass into the bloodstream. Although the bite is usually painless, it may cause swelling.

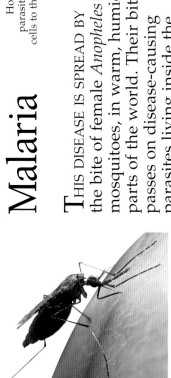

3 IN THE BLOODSTREAM
Newly emerged adult parasites start travelling through the infected person's blood.

PROTECT YOURSELF AGAINST MOSQUITOES
YOU OWE IT TO YOURSELF YOUR COMRADES YOUR EFFICIENCY

HELPING PEOPLE TO HELP THEMSELVES
Poster campaigns have proved to be a vital tool in the fight against malaria. Publicity is essential, as cases have been rising steadily since the early 1960s. This was a time when the disease started to reappear, just when many people thought it was no longer a serious threat. Malaria has reappeared partly because poor countries have not been able to afford expensive healthcare. Also, people travelling abroad from richer countries often fail to take the threat of malaria seriously.

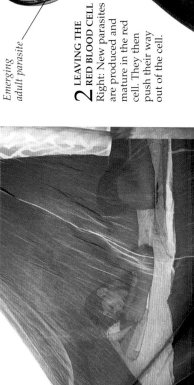
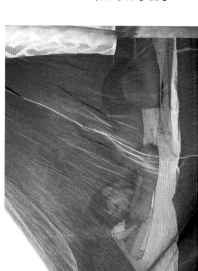

Red blood cell

Emerging adult parasite

2 LEAVING THE RED BLOOD CELL
Right: New parasites are produced and mature in the red cell. They then push their way out of the cell.

MOSQUITO NET
In areas where malaria is common, people sleep under fine nets to protect themselves from being bitten. If the nets are soaked in an insecticide that kills the mosquitoes, then this further reduces the risk of infection. Mosquitoes feed at night, so it is important to close windows, or fit fine metal screens over open windows. People who are outside at night should cover up as much as possible. They should also apply special repellent on any exposed skin.

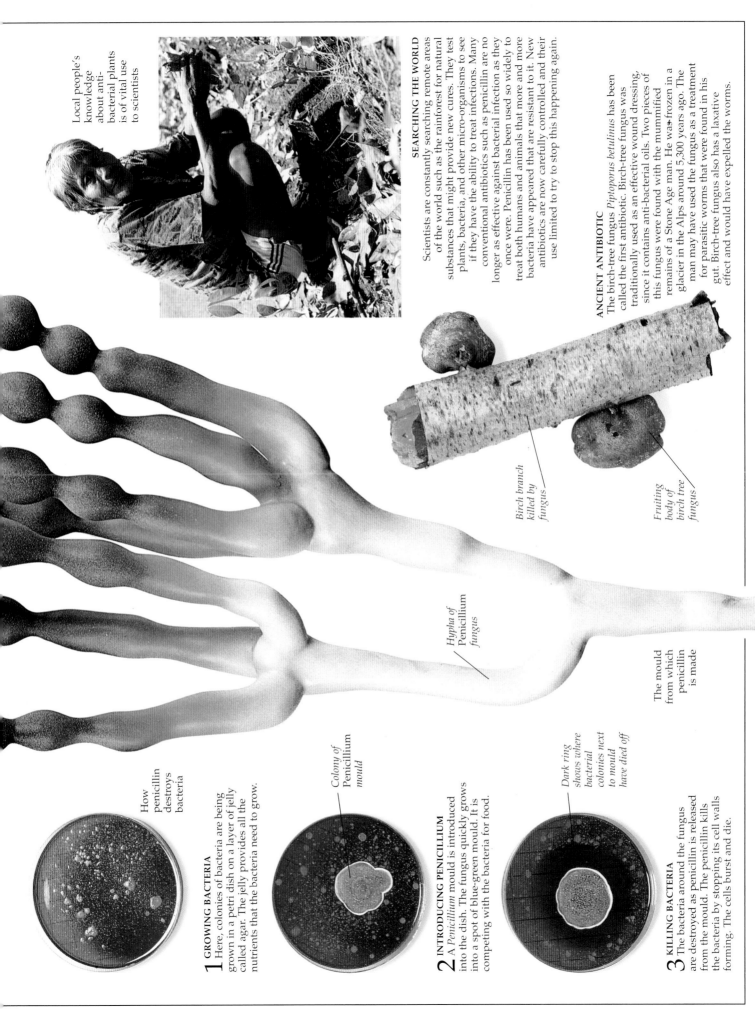

Local people's knowledge about anti-bacterial plants is of vital use to scientists

SEARCHING THE WORLD

Scientists are constantly searching remote areas of the world such as the rainforest for natural substances that might provide new cures. They test plants, bacteria, and other micro-organisms to see if they have the ability to treat infections. Many conventional antibiotics such as penicillin are no longer as effective against bacterial infection as they once were. Penicillin has been used so widely to treat both humans and animals that more and more bacteria have appeared that are resistant to it. New antibiotics are now carefully controlled and their use limited to try to stop this happening again.

ANCIENT ANTIBIOTIC

The birch-tree fungus *Piptoporus betulinus* has been called the first antibiotic. Birch-tree fungus was traditionally used as an effective wound dressing, since it contains anti-bacterial oils. Two pieces of this fungus were found with the mummified remains of a Stone Age man. He was frozen in a glacier in the Alps around 5,300 years ago. The man may have used the fungus as a treatment for parasitic worms that were found in his gut. Birch-tree fungus also has a laxative effect and would have expelled the worms.

Birch branch killed by fungus

Fruiting body of birch tree fungus

Hypha of Penicillium fungus

The mould from which penicillin is made

How penicillin destroys bacteria

1 GROWING BACTERIA
Here, colonies of bacteria are being grown in a petri dish on a layer of jelly called agar. The jelly provides all the nutrients that the bacteria need to grow.

Colony of Penicillium mould

2 INTRODUCING PENICILLIUM
A *Penicillium* mould is introduced into the dish. The fungus quickly grows into a spot of blue-green mould. It is competing with the bacteria for food.

Dark ring shows where bacterial colonies next to mould have died off

3 KILLING BACTERIA
The bacteria around the fungus are destroyed as penicillin is released from the mould. The penicillin kills the bacteria by stopping its cell walls forming. The cells burst and die.

Nature's medicine cabinet

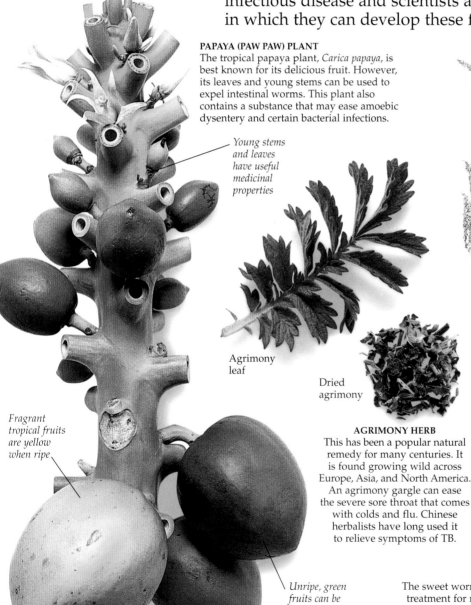

Page from a medieval herbal manuscript

FOR THOUSANDS OF YEARS, plant-based remedies were the only form of treatment available for most diseases. This situation continued right into the 1900s, when scientists started making drugs artificially and herbal medicine declined in importance. From around the 1970s, interest turned back to plants. It was realized that there might be all kinds of "undiscovered" substances in plants and fungi that could be used in new drugs. Scientists now routinely screen plants for medical properties. They also look closely at traditional plant remedies used by different native peoples all over the world. Exciting advances have been made. It seems that various plants can help in the fight against infectious disease and scientists are looking at ways in which they can develop these for widespread use.

PAPAYA (PAW PAW) PLANT
The tropical papaya plant, *Carica papaya*, is best known for its delicious fruit. However, its leaves and young stems can be used to expel intestinal worms. This plant also contains a substance that may ease amoebic dysentery and certain bacterial infections.

Young stems and leaves have useful medicinal properties

Fragrant tropical fruits are yellow when ripe

Unripe, green fruits can be eaten as a vegetable

Agrimony leaf

Dried agrimony

AGRIMONY HERB
This has been a popular natural remedy for many centuries. It is found growing wild across Europe, Asia, and North America. An agrimony gargle can ease the severe sore throat that comes with colds and flu. Chinese herbalists have long used it to relieve symptoms of TB.

Dried branches of sweet wormwood, *Artemisia annua*

SWEET WORMWOOD BUSH
The sweet wormwood plant is a traditional Chinese treatment for malaria. In the late 20th century, when malaria began to resist modern drugs, scientists examined this plant more closely. They isolated powerful anti-malaria substances called artemisinins. Drugs based on these substances are now widely used around the world.

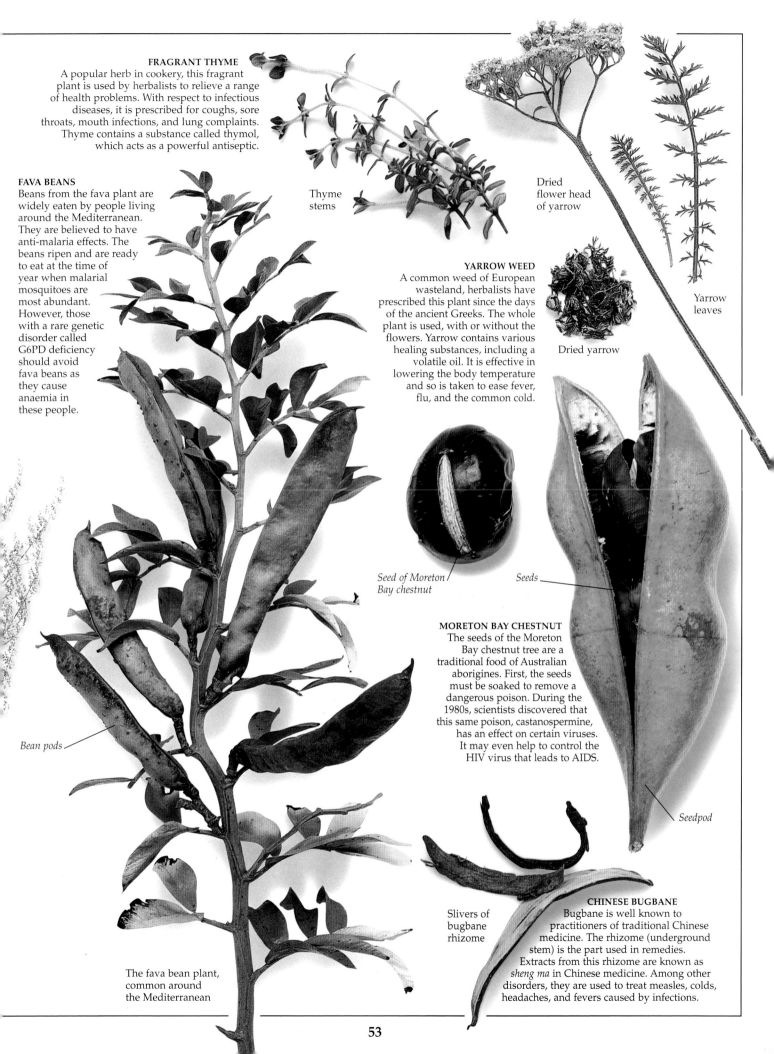

FRAGRANT THYME
A popular herb in cookery, this fragrant plant is used by herbalists to relieve a range of health problems. With respect to infectious diseases, it is prescribed for coughs, sore throats, mouth infections, and lung complaints. Thyme contains a substance called thymol, which acts as a powerful antiseptic.

Thyme stems

Dried flower head of yarrow

Yarrow leaves

FAVA BEANS
Beans from the fava plant are widely eaten by people living around the Mediterranean. They are believed to have anti-malaria effects. The beans ripen and are ready to eat at the time of year when malarial mosquitoes are most abundant. However, those with a rare genetic disorder called G6PD deficiency should avoid fava beans as they cause anaemia in these people.

YARROW WEED
A common weed of European wasteland, herbalists have prescribed this plant since the days of the ancient Greeks. The whole plant is used, with or without the flowers. Yarrow contains various healing substances, including a volatile oil. It is effective in lowering the body temperature and so is taken to ease fever, flu, and the common cold.

Dried yarrow

Seed of Moreton Bay chestnut

Seeds

MORETON BAY CHESTNUT
The seeds of the Moreton Bay chestnut tree are a traditional food of Australian aborigines. First, the seeds must be soaked to remove a dangerous poison. During the 1980s, scientists discovered that this same poison, castanospermine, has an effect on certain viruses. It may even help to control the HIV virus that leads to AIDS.

Bean pods

Seedpod

Slivers of bugbane rhizome

CHINESE BUGBANE
Bugbane is well known to practitioners of traditional Chinese medicine. The rhizome (underground stem) is the part used in remedies. Extracts from this rhizome are known as *sheng ma* in Chinese medicine. Among other disorders, they are used to treat measles, colds, headaches, and fevers caused by infections.

The fava bean plant, common around the Mediterranean

53

Animal plagues

EPIDEMICS ALSO STRIKE the animal world. Animals normally develop some immunity to diseases that are common in their region. However, if they are weakened by factors such as starvation, then these diseases can take a hold. Severe epidemics also break out among livestock. This usually occurs when they are introduced into new areas where they have no immunity to the diseases carried by wild animals already living there. Animal infection is controlled by quarantine and slaughter. If livestock has been affected by a locally common disease, they often need to be vaccinated against infection.

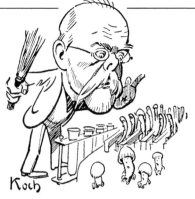

ROBERT KOCH
This comical cartoon from 1910 shows the pioneering German bacteriologist Robert Koch (1843–1910) "lecturing" his laboratory samples. Koch was the first person to show the causes of anthrax and rinderpest. He also developed a vaccine to protect livestock from rinderpest.

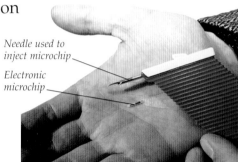

Needle used to inject microchip

Electronic microchip

TAGGING ANIMALS WITH MICROCHIPS
Tiny microchips can be inserted under animals' skin. This identifies them if they are captured and allows their movements to be tracked. Tags can also be used to identify pets that have been vaccinated against diseases such as rabies. This means they do not need to be held in quarantine.

SAVING THE SERENGETI LIONS
Here, a vet in Tanzania, East Africa, fits a radio collar to a lion. In the mid-1990s, around 1,000 lions on the East African Serengeti Plain died from the feverish viral disease, distemper. They probably caught it from wild dogs. Monitoring the movements of lions in the area with radio collars enabled experts to follow the spread of the disease. The distemper vanished of its own accord as surviving lions became immune.

ANIMALS ON THE AFRICAN PLAINS
Wildlife on the African plains has suffered a range of diseases. Rinderpest is a very infectious viral illness that causes total physical breakdown. It has affected various animals, including wild buffalo, antelope, and domestic cattle. The disease has been controlled by vaccination and slaughter of animals.

A mystery disease that paralyzes elephant trunks appeared in the 1990s

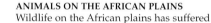

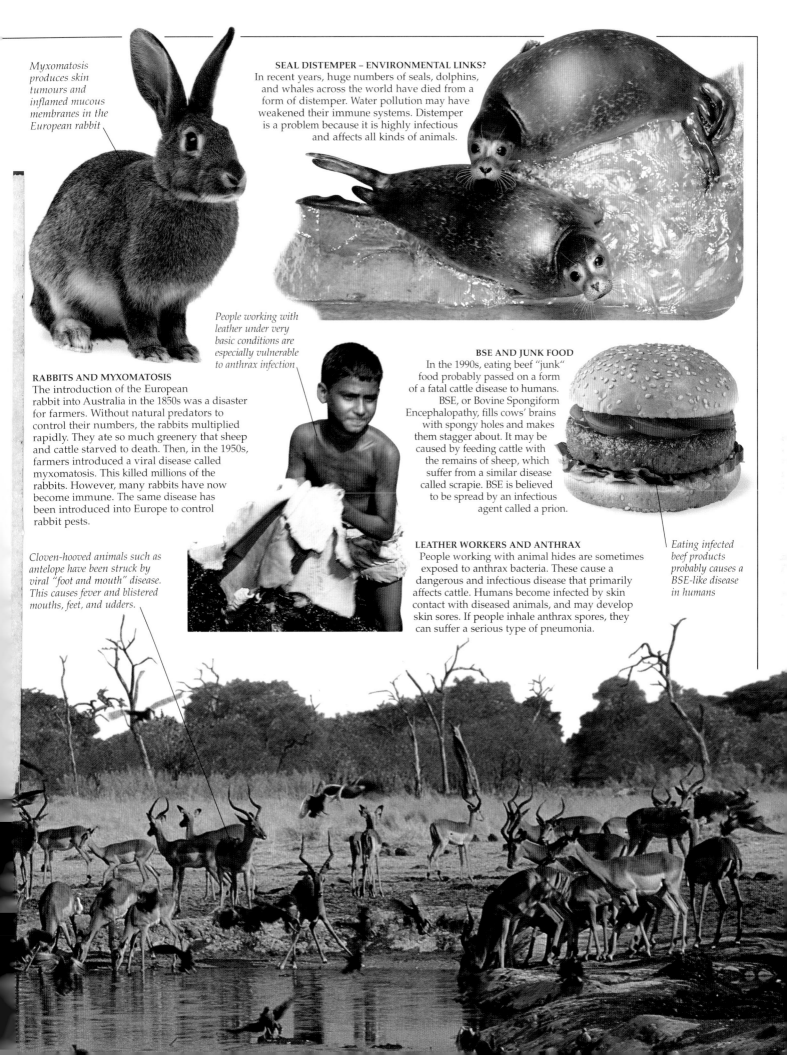

Myxomatosis produces skin tumours and inflamed mucous membranes in the European rabbit

SEAL DISTEMPER – ENVIRONMENTAL LINKS?
In recent years, huge numbers of seals, dolphins, and whales across the world have died from a form of distemper. Water pollution may have weakened their immune systems. Distemper is a problem because it is highly infectious and affects all kinds of animals.

People working with leather under very basic conditions are especially vulnerable to anthrax infection

RABBITS AND MYXOMATOSIS
The introduction of the European rabbit into Australia in the 1850s was a disaster for farmers. Without natural predators to control their numbers, the rabbits multiplied rapidly. They ate so much greenery that sheep and cattle starved to death. Then, in the 1950s, farmers introduced a viral disease called myxomatosis. This killed millions of the rabbits. However, many rabbits have now become immune. The same disease has been introduced into Europe to control rabbit pests.

BSE AND JUNK FOOD
In the 1990s, eating beef "junk" food probably passed on a form of a fatal cattle disease to humans. BSE, or Bovine Spongiform Encephalopathy, fills cows' brains with spongy holes and makes them stagger about. It may be caused by feeding cattle with the remains of sheep, which suffer from a similar disease called scrapie. BSE is believed to be spread by an infectious agent called a prion.

Cloven-hooved animals such as antelope have been struck by viral "foot and mouth" disease. This causes fever and blistered mouths, feet, and udders.

LEATHER WORKERS AND ANTHRAX
People working with animal hides are sometimes exposed to anthrax bacteria. These cause a dangerous and infectious disease that primarily affects cattle. Humans become infected by skin contact with diseased animals, and may develop skin sores. If people inhale anthrax spores, they can suffer a serious type of pneumonia.

Eating infected beef products probably causes a BSE-like disease in humans

Hot viruses and superbugs

NEW BUGS ARE EMERGING that resist attack by drugs or our immune system. Some produce illnesses that we have not met before. Others are new, highly resistant forms of familiar microbes, and can even be caught in modern hospitals. Drug-resistant "superbug" bacteria cause some of the problems. However, most are caused by so-called "hot" viruses that normally only affect certain animals, and to which we have no immunity. People may be catching these viruses because the human population is expanding and clearing animal habitats for farming and housing, bringing humans and animals into closer contact. Fortunately, most animal bugs are poorly adapted to living in humans and so far have caused no major epidemics.

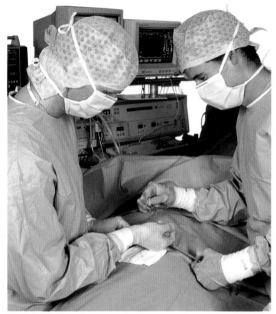

HOSPITAL SUPERBUGS
Some of the new diseases are developing within hospitals. One is called MRSA (Methicillin-Resistant Staphylococcus Aureus). *S. aureus* is a bacterium that is found on the skin. Recently, some strains have developed resistance to even the strongest antibiotics. They can spread rapidly among hospital patients, weakened by illness. Experts are making sure that hospitals are as clean as possible, as careless cleaning practices may also be a factor.

TAKING PROPER PRECAUTIONS
When highly infectious "new" bugs cause disease outbreaks, victims' bodies must be buried correctly by equipped personnel in order to prevent the microbes from spreading further. WHO (the World Health Organization) monitors outbreaks of these diseases closely and sends trained teams to take control of the situation.

INFORMING THE PUBLIC
Posters have been displayed in areas where diseases like Ebola fever have previously broken out. Their job is to explain what people must do if the disease breaks out again.

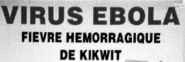

Contact with infected blood must be avoided. This is how the Ebola virus has usually been spread

Poster used in a French-speaking part of Africa

The bodies of victims should not be washed by untrained people. This custom has spread the Ebola virus to relatives in the past

All used syringes, which might contain infected blood, have to be destroyed

Victims' clothing is burned, in order to kill any microbes

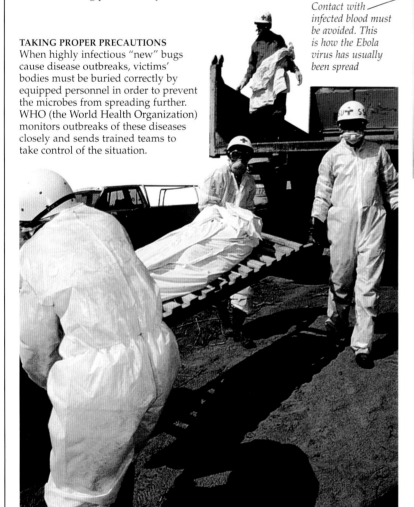

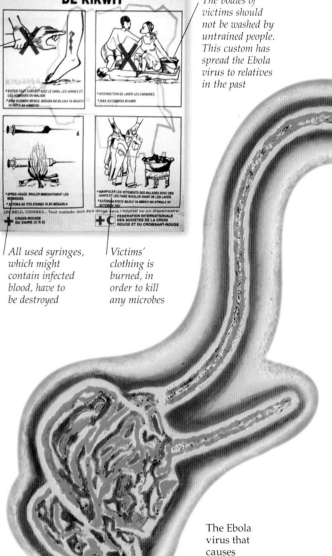

The Ebola virus that causes Ebola fever

EBOLA VIRUS

The Ebola virus can cause a high fever, rashes, and severe internal and external bleeding. It may be fatal. The virus is named after the Ebola River in central Africa. The first outbreaks among humans were recorded there in 1976. Since then, there have been several more in Africa, as well as outbreaks among primates. It is not known how the virus gets into human bodies, or how it attacks cells, although we do know that it can be spread via contact with the body fluids of infected people. The virus may produce proteins that hinder the human immune system, allowing the virus to reproduce rapidly.

A single Ebola virus, looping back on itself

Long, thread-like shape

African grassland monkeys

SHOWERHEADS AND LEGIONNAIRE'S DISEASE

Showerheads are one of the places that the bacteria that cause Legionnaire's disease – *Legionella pneumophilia* – gather. This is because the bacteria breed in hot water and are spread in water droplets. Other common breeding sites for the bacteria include air conditioning and ventilation systems found in hotels and office blocks. These all use water and this explains why large numbers of people often fall ill at the same time, in the same place.

THE STORY BEHIND LEGIONNAIRE'S DISEASE

The American Legion – a military veterans' organization – has given Legionnaire's disease its distinctive name. In 1976, a meeting of the American Legion was held in Philadelphia, USA. Many of the delegates stayed in one hotel, and soon they became ill with a flu-like disease that turned into pneumonia. Several died. Since then, much has been learned about the disease and where it strikes. It can be treated with antibiotics.

The small Mastomys *rat commonly lives in and around people's homes in West Africa*

MARBURG DISEASE

This viral disease first appeared in Europe in 1967, among laboratory workers in Marburg, Germany and in Yugoslavia. The technicians had been working with cells taken from green monkeys, found on the African grasslands. Since then, more human cases have occurred, all with an African link. The virus and its disease are similar to Ebola. Like Ebola, few facts are known about Marburg.

LASSA FEVER CARRIER

This rat was found to be the cause of a "new" disease outbreak in Nigeria, Africa, in 1969. The disease was named Lassa fever, and its symptoms were much like Ebola. There have been several African outbreaks since then. *Mastomys* rats are often infected by the Lassa virus, and excrete it in their urine. Humans catch the virus if they come into contact with urine or droppings, in bedding for example.

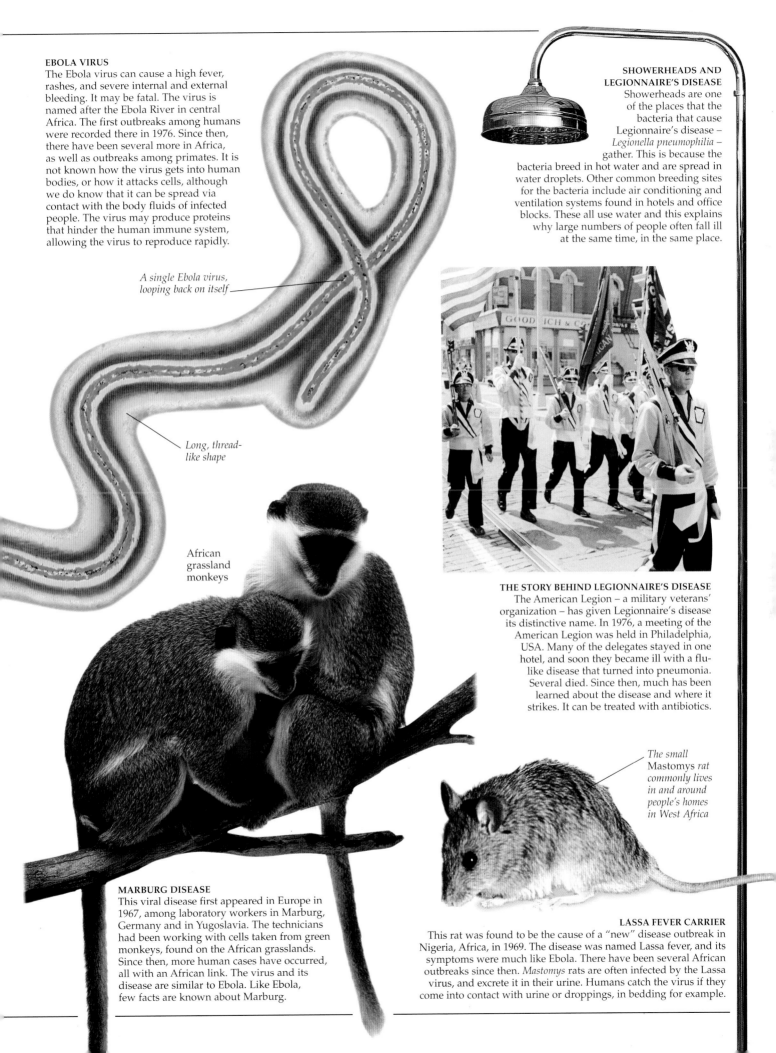

HIV and AIDS

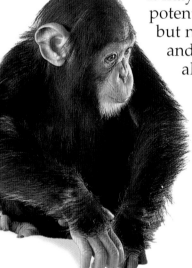

The HIV viruses that can lead to full-blown AIDS

In the early 1980s, mysterious outbreaks of pneumonia and rare cancers appeared in the USA. These were the first signs of AIDS, a new disease with no obvious cause. It spread rapidly, and there were frantic efforts to find its origins. By 1985 it was pandemic in the USA and Africa, and by 1990 it affected the whole world. The cause of AIDS is infection with HIV (Human Immunodeficiency Virus), which attacks the immune system. The virus is spread by contact with infected blood and body fluids – mostly through sexual intercourse and sharing needles. Infection leaves the body vulnerable to attack from conditions that would not usually turn into serious problems. A group of diseases such as pneumonia develop and these are called AIDS – Acquired Immunodeficiency Syndrome. HIV cannot be dislodged from the body's cells. Though it may lie dormant for a long time, it eventually causes potentially fatal disease. No cure has been found, but new drugs stop the virus from reproducing and allow those infected to live almost normal lives.

How HIV infects a human T-cell

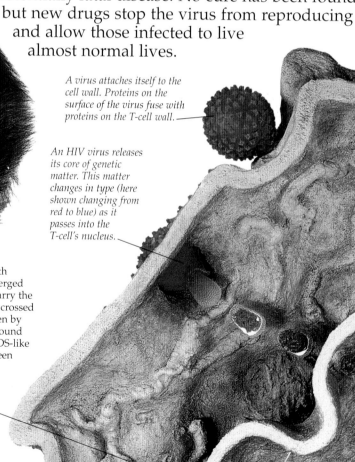

A virus attaches itself to the cell wall. Proteins on the surface of the virus fuse with proteins on the T-cell wall.

An HIV virus releases its core of genetic matter. This matter changes in type (here shown changing from red to blue) as it passes into the T-cell's nucleus.

Nucleus of T-cell

MYSTERIOUS ORIGINS
The origins of HIV have been linked with chimpanzees. Some think that AIDS emerged from African chimpanzees, which can carry the virus without becoming ill. It may have crossed to humans when chimpanzees were eaten by hunters. Similar types of virus are also found in cats, and cats go on to develop an AIDS-like disease. The original source has never been found, although research continues.

ATTACKING THE IMMUNE SYSTEM
Here, an HIV virus is breaking into a human T-cell. These cells are part of the body's immune system, used normally to fight all kinds of infection. Once inside the cell, the virus releases its genetic material. This finds its way to the nucleus of the T-cell and alters the T-cell's genetic material. As the virus takes over the T-cell, the cell starts to produce viral genetic material. This travels out of the nucleus and whole new viruses are assembled – the virus is reproducing.

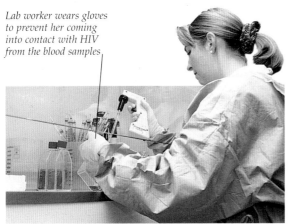

Lab worker wears gloves to prevent her coming into contact with HIV from the blood samples

THE SYRINGE LINK

Syringes are a common way of spreading HIV. People who inject drugs and share their syringes with others can easily spread the virus. Also, if people use syringes for medical purposes such as vaccinations, and the same syringe is used for many people, disease can spread. Medical people now use fresh, disposable syringes for each person. Similarly, distributing free disposable syringes to drug-abusers has done much to control HIV.

LABORATORY RESEARCH

Laboratory tests have been devised to show the presence of the HIV virus in human body fluids. If people know that they have the virus, they can take measures that stop them from spreading it accidentally to others. These tests are especially important for pregnant women carrying HIV, as they might pass it to their unborn child. If the virus is detected in the mother, treatment can be given to prevent the baby from becoming infected.

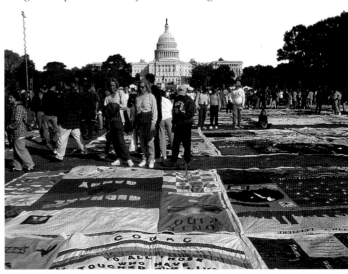

HIV COMMEMORATIVE QUILT

This giant quilt was designed to remember some of those who had died from AIDs. Here, it is on show for the first time on the Mall, Washington DC, USA, in 1987. Each square of the quilt represents an individual or a group of people who have died. The squares were sewn by friends and families of the patients. Many other such quilts have been produced all over the world, helping to raise awareness of this modern disease.

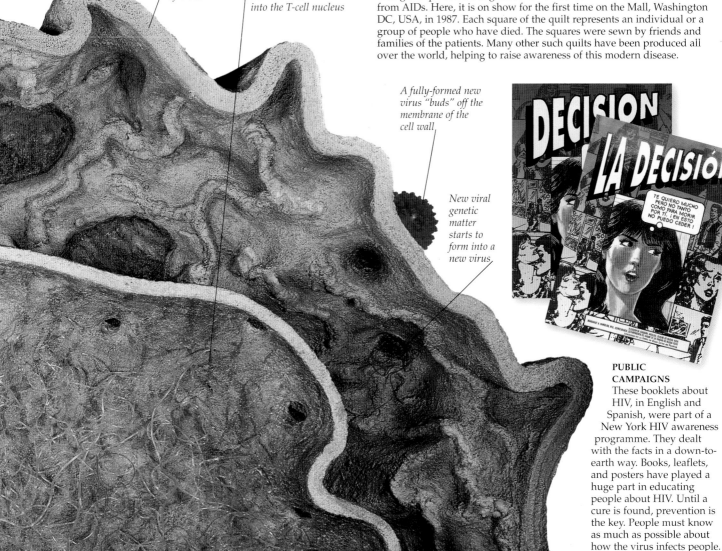

Membrane of T-cell

Viral genetic matter (red strands) inserted into the T-cell nucleus

A fully-formed new virus "buds" off the membrane of the cell wall

New viral genetic matter starts to form into a new virus

PUBLIC CAMPAIGNS

These booklets about HIV, in English and Spanish, were part of a New York HIV awareness programme. They dealt with the facts in a down-to-earth way. Books, leaflets, and posters have played a huge part in educating people about HIV. Until a cure is found, prevention is the key. People must know as much as possible about how the virus infects people.

Germ warfare

THIS EXPRESSION REFERS to deliberate attempts to weaken whole populations of people by infecting them, or their livestock or crops, with disease. Forms of germ warfare have existed for many centuries. Plague-infested bodies were used to spread disease among the enemy in the Middle Ages. In the 1700s, whole tribes of Native Americans in modern-day Canada were wiped out by smallpox caught from infected blankets given to them by the British. In recent years, germ warfare has been threatened but never used on a large scale. The idea is for a country to develop strains of microbes that are easily spread, while its own troops are protected by vaccination. Germ warfare is prohibited by international conventions as one of the greatest risks to human life. Research is only allowed into methods of protection against possible germ attack.

Skull and crossbones symbolize poisonous substances

KEEP AWAY!
A black-bordered yellow triangle is a general international warning symbol. With a skull and crossbones on it, it is a warning about toxic substances. In the event of a germ outbreak, a large area might have to have warning signs posted for a long time afterwards.

Siege of Nicaea, 1098

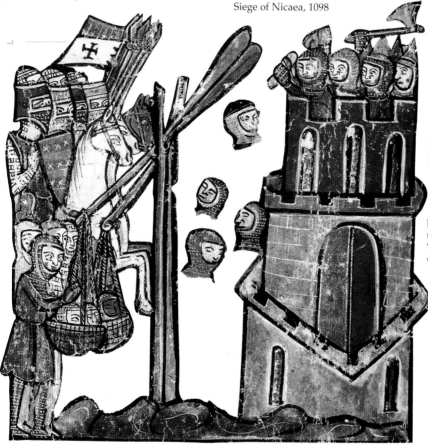

EARLY FORMS OF GERM WARFARE
In 1098, Crusader armies besieging Nicaea (now Iznik, in Turkey) are said to have catapulted diseased human heads into the city in order to spread disease. Mongol soldiers attacking the Black Sea port of Kaffa, in the 1300s, apparently did the same with plague-infected bodies. (This helped to set off the Black Death that ravaged Europe during the Middle Ages.) The Russians are said to have used the same weapon against the Swedes in the 18th century.

Sealed suit to protect against contamination

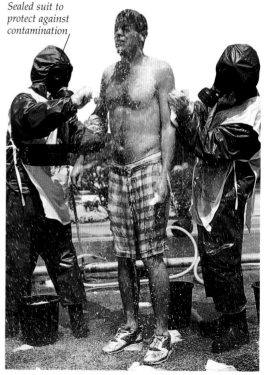

ANTHRAX WARFARE
This picture shows anthrax bacteria in a human lung. Anthrax is one of the microbes that have been considered for use in germ warfare. Normally a disease of livestock, anthrax in humans can cause either skin ulceration or pneumonia. Anthrax also forms spores that can persist in the soil for many years, so if used in warfare it could make an area permanently uninhabitable.

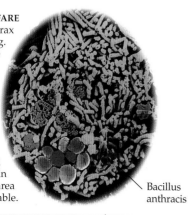

Bacillus anthracis

THE GULF WAR
Here, a soldier fighting in the Gulf War (1990–91) is given a very thorough decontaminating wash. This international war broke out when Iraq invaded Kuwait, in the Middle East. The Western nations involved feared the use of chemical and bacteriological weapons by Iraq. Some chemical weapons were in fact used, but they had no serious effects.

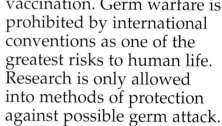

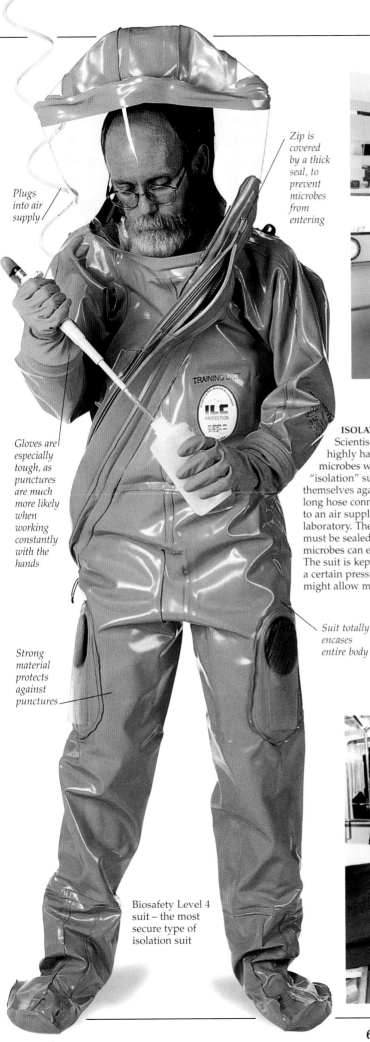

Plugs into air supply

Zip is covered by a thick seal, to prevent microbes from entering

Gloves are especially tough, as punctures are much more likely when working constantly with the hands

Strong material protects against punctures

Suit totally encases entire body

Biosafety Level 4 suit – the most secure type of isolation suit

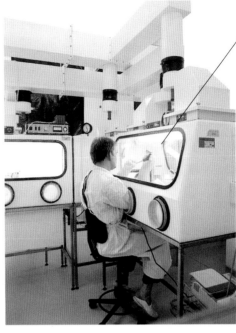

Researchers working within these special sealed cabinets do not need to wear full safety suits like the one on the left

GERM LABORATORIES

High-security laboratories are equipped so that researchers can work with dangerous bacteria and viruses as safely as possible. The organisms are often handled inside cabinets, with the laboratory worker wearing long protective gloves. The air inside the cabinet is kept at a special reduced pressure and is constantly extracted and filtered. Any work on producing germs for germ warfare would be carried out in this type of laboratory.

ISOLATION SUIT

Scientists researching highly hazardous microbes wear special "isolation" suits to protect themselves against infection. A long hose connects the wearer to an air supply unit in the laboratory. The air supply must be sealed off so that no microbes can enter the suit. The suit is kept constantly at a certain pressure, as changes might allow microbes to enter.

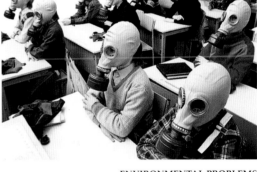

ENVIRONMENTAL PROBLEMS

These children, from Ventspils in Latvia, are practising how to use gas masks. The masks filter out dangerous microbes and must be worn once the air we breathe becomes contaminated. There have been severe problems around Ventspils because the air and water have become severely tainted with industrial waste. If people were planning a germ attack, contaminating the water would be an effective way of causing rapid damage.

Workers dressed in safety suits and gas masks

JAPANESE ATTACK

Here, workers decontaminate subway trains in Tokyo, Japan. In 1995, commuters on the subway were attacked with "nerve gas" (so-called because it affects the nerves). Fortunately, few people died. The gas used was one that had been developed in Germany in World War II. The leader of a Japanese religious cult called Aum was charged with making the attack.

The continuing war

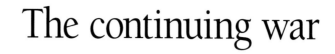

EXPLORING GENETIC LINKS
The cells of every living thing, including bacteria and viruses, contain information about that organism in a chemical form called DNA. Researchers are now studying the DNA of microbes in order to discover exactly how they attack the body, and why they often become resistant to drugs.

Oᴜʀ ᴡᴀʀ ᴀɢᴀɪɴꜱᴛ ᴇᴘɪᴅᴇᴍɪᴄꜱ is not over yet, but new advances are made all the time. The most extraordinary achievements of recent years have been the mass-vaccination programmes. These have done much to reduce diseases such as polio, and to eradicate human smallpox altogether. The best strategy we have is keeping a step ahead. Environmental changes and disease patterns are now tracked very closely in order to predict disease outbreaks. We have also realized that effective treatments come in many forms. Costly drugs may prevent many deaths, but simple measures such as giving lost salts to children weakened by diarrhoea also saves huge numbers of lives each year.

Model of part of a DNA molecule

Image created with two satellites

Surface proteins

HANTAVIRUS INFECTION – ONE OF THE "NEW" DISEASES
This shows a type of hantavirus, which can cause severe symptoms such as pneumonia and liver failure. The virus is spread by contact with rodent droppings. Hantaviruses are among the disease-causing microbes that have suddenly "appeared" in recent years. Illness is rare, and scientists have already discovered that simple measures to keep rodents away can do much to limit the risk of an epidemic.

Computer-generated satellite map

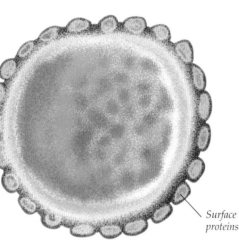

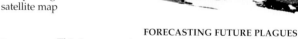

FORECASTING FUTURE PLAGUES
This is a computer-manipulated version of an image produced by satellites set up to survey the Earth from space. Such images may reveal details that help experts to predict where and when disease outbreaks might occur. For example, weather satellites can identify changes that affect insect populations. An increase in damp conditions causes mosquitoes to breed rapidly, which can lead to more outbreaks of malaria and yellow fever.

GETTING HEALTH AID TO REMOTE AREAS
Here, a team of French aid workers has just flown supplies into a remote part of Cambodia, Southeast Asia. Much of the hope for the future lies with agencies like this, which can treat people on the spot. They are increasing in number and attract highly skilled medical professionals.

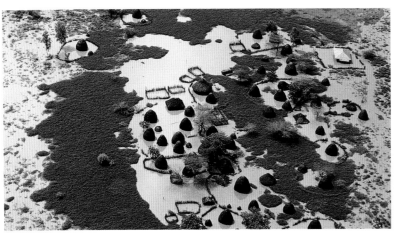

NATURAL DISASTERS AND DISEASE – NEW WAYS OF COPING
This ariel view of the Tana River Valley in Kenya, Africa, shows severe flooding caused by torrential rain. Major floods often bring people into contact with sewage, and drinking water becomes contaminated with dead animals that have drowned. The result is often epidemics such as food poisoning, typhoid, and cholera. International efforts are being made to control flooding. This is done with dams and with massive tree-planting programmes, which can slow the progress of water rushing down from mountains to the lowlands.

CHANGING PEOPLE'S HABITS
Simply getting people to follow basic hygiene rules makes a huge difference. Washing your hands after using the toilet and before preparing food is the best way to reduce infections that cause diarrhoea. Many areas still have no access to clean washing and drinking water. Aid agencies are working hard to provide wells in these regions.

AIDS poster from Senegal, West Africa

Poster promoting immunization of babies and toddlers, from Nepal

बच्चालाई बेलैमा खोप दिलाऔं
रोग लाग्नबाट जोगाऔं

खोपको
सेवा र सल्लाहका लागि

STOP SIDA

SIDA

PENSEZ-Y
SERVICE DE L'EDUCATION POUR LA SANTE · M.S.H.·C.N.P.S.·SENEGAL

EXPLAINING THE ISSUES
Public health campaigns, using posters and leaflets, must be simple, as many communities around the world have few reading skills. Campaigns advising mothers how to re-hydrate babies suffering from diarrhoea have proved highly successful, and there are hopes that HIV programmes will do just as well.

Holder for vaccine

VACCINATION PROGRAMMES
"Guns" like this have been used for some of the highly successful mass-vaccination programmes of recent years. Today, widespread vaccination is as important as ever. Simpler, disposable syringes now tend to be used rather than guns.

Injection head, which fires vaccine into skin under high pressure

Trigger

Multiple-shot gun for large-scale innoculation

TREATMENT FOR ALL
These Amazonian people from South America are being given a vaccine orally (by mouth). Doctors are experimenting with giving people vaccines via mouth drops or nasal sprays. These methods do not involve injections, which have to be managed with care in order to avoid infection and which some people find offputting. Research is constantly underway to find as many new, easy ways of getting vaccines to people as possible.

Index

Acknowledgements

Dorling Kindersley would like to thank:

All involved at the AMNH for their patient help, in particular: Dr Rob DeSalle, Curator; Maron L Waxman, Director, Special Publishing; Kathryn McGinley, Coordinator, Special Publishing; Larry Langham, AMNH's *Epidemic* exhibition designer; David Harvey, Exhibition Director; and others listed elsewhere. Sheila Collins, Laura Roberts, and Simon Holland for design and editorial assistance. To West One for the showerhead picture, 57r.
Index: Chris Bernstein.
Illustrator: Joanna Cameron.
Model-makers: Chris Reynolds, BBC (40tl); Peter Minister (40r); the AMNH microbe models: James Stoop and Barrett Klein.
DK photography: Peter Anderson, Geoff Brightling, Jane Burton, Andy Crawford, Geoff Dann, Jake Fitzjones, Steve Gorton, Frank Greenaway, Dave King, Susanna Price, Jules Selmes, James Stevenson, Clive Streeter, Harry Taylor, Jerry Young (31t, 57bl), Science Museum photographers: David Exton, John Lepine.

The publisher would like to thank the following for their kind permission to reproduce their photographs:
a=above, b=below, c=centre, l-left, r=right, t=top:

AKG London: 13r. Ardea London Ltd: P. Morris 57br. Associated Press: NTB 35cr. Dr. Edward C. Atwater, AIDS Education Archive: 63cr (far). Barnaby's Picture Library: Colin Underhill 31cl. BBC Natural History Unit:

Charlie Hamilton James 31bl. Bridgeman Art Library, London / New York: Bibliotheque Nationale, France Crusaders bombard Nicaea with heads c.1098, by William of Tyre (c.1130-85) Estoire d'Outremer, (12th century) 60cl; Central Saint Martin's College of Art and Design, London, UK Over London – By Rail, from 'London, a Pilgrimage', written by William Blanchard Jerrold (1826-94), engraved by Stephane Pannemaker (1847-1930), pub. 1872 (engraving) by Gustave Doré (1832-83) (after) 16tl; Library of Congress, Washington D.C., USA The First Landing of Columbus on the Shores of the New World at San Salvador, Oct. 12th 1492 by D. Puebla, pub. by Currier and Ives 10b; Musee Condé, Chantilly, France/Giraudon Nathan shows War, Plague and Death to King David Hours of Nicolas Le Camus, (Late 15th c.) 13cl; Musée d'Orsay, Paris, France/Lauros-Giraudon Louis Pasteur (1822-95) in his Laboratory, 1885 (oil on canvas) by Albert Gustaf Aristides Edelfelt (1854-1905) 14tl; Museo di San Marco dell'Angelico, Florence, Italy Historiated initial 'O' depicting Aegidius (St. Giles) (d.c.700) enthroned surrounded by angels, 1421 (vellum) Messale di Sant'Egidio, (1421) 26tl; Private Collection The Seven Plagues of Egypt; Moses and the plague of boils (printed book) Nuremberg Bible (Biblia Sacra Germanaica), (1483) 6tr; Private Collection/Chris Beetles, London "Until they came to the River Weser, wherein all plunged in", illustration from 'The Pied Piper of Hamelin', 1912 (w/c, pencil on paper) by Margaret Tarrant (1888-1959) 12c;

Private Collection/Roger-Viollet, Paris The First War of the Balkans: Cholera Epidemic, from 'Le Petit Journal', 1st December 1912 (litho) by French School (20th century) 22tl. British Library, London: 52tl. BT Museum: 35ca. Corbis UK Ltd: Bettmann 16bl, 30tl, 34cl, 35tr; C. Moore 11cl; Lee Snider 59tr; Owen Franken 19cr; Steve Raymer 36tr, 39cl; The Purcell Team 44bc; Tim Page 62b. Sue Cunningham Photographic: 9br, 26br, 37tr. Environmental Images: Herbert Girardet 51tr; Leslie Garland 25cl; Robert Brook 43b; Sue Cunningham 47br. The Art Archive: 22-23; Academie de Medecine Paris 28bl; British Museum 28tl; Private Collection 38tl. Mary Evans Picture Library: 10tr, 12b, 13tc, 24bl, 26bl, 27tl, 28r, 34tl, 49bc. Ronald Grant Archive: Columbia Pictures 37tl. Hulton Getty: 11cr, 21br, 23tc, 38-39, 45cla. Hutchison Library: 29cl; Jesco Von Puttkamer 63bl. Museum Of London: 13tl. N.A.S.A.: 62–63. N.H.P.A.: Christopher Ratier 54cl; Martin Harvery 54-55. Oxford Scientific Films: Paul McCullagh 44clb. Panos Pictures: Caroline Penn 39tr; Giacomo Pirozzi 39br. Powerstock Photolibrary / Zefa: William Bernard 30b. Rex Features: 54tr, 61br; Aivars Liepins/AFI 61cr; Albert Facelly 17crb; John Le Fevre 56cr, 56bl; Jonathan Shaul 60br. Science & Society Picture Library: 11l, 13c; Science Museum: London 17b, 22bl, 23c, 24cl, 24crb, 24-25, 29tl, 29tc, 29tr, 63br. Science Photo Library: 27tr, 42cl, 62cl; A. B. Dowsett 39cr, 60bl; A. Crump, TDR, WHO 27ca; Alfred Pasieka 36bl; Barry Dowsett 56-57; Bernard Pierre Wolff 29bl; BSIP Laurent 59tl; BSIP VEM 15r; CDC 9tl, 35br; Chris Priest & Mark Clarke 38c; CNRI 41b, 50tr; Custom Medical Stock Photo 48bc; Dr Jeremy Burgess 40bl; Dr P.

Marazzi 41tr, 43cl; Dr P. Marazzi 40cl; Dr Rosalind King 26-27; Dr. Karl Lounatmaa 19tl; Eye of Science 29br; Geoff Tompkinson 32bl; Institut Pasteur/CNRI 17tl; James King-Holmes 61tr; John Bavosi 45bc; John Burbidge 12cla; John Hadfield 48bl; London School of Hygiene and Tropical Medicine 21cr; Martin Dohrn 32bc; Matt Meadows, Peter Arnold Inc 33tr; Microfield Scientific Ltd 49tl; Mike Peres/Custom Medical Stock Photo 43crb; NASA 15cla; National Library of Medicine 50cl; NIBSC 8br, 39tc; Philippe Plailly/Eurelios 31br; Simon Fraser 7bl, 56tl; Simon Fraser/Royal Victoria Infirmary, Newcastle-Upon-Tyne 36-37, 37br; Sinclair Stammers 46bl; Stevie Grand 42bl. Still Pictures: G. Griffiths, Christian Aid 63tl; Julio Etchart 17tr; Mark Edwards 9tr, 9cr, 23crb, 46crb; Martin Specht 17cr; Shehzad Noorani 47bl, 55cl. Tony Stone Images: Alan Wycheck 11b; Paul Chesley 7tc. UNICEF: 63c (near). The Wellcome Institute Library, London: 16c, 33br, 44cl, 46tl. Wilberforce House, Hull City Museums: 11t.

Jacket:

AKG London: inside front tr. The Art Archive: Private Collection back br. Bridgeman Art Library, London / New York: Private Collection/Roger-Viollet, Paris The First War of the Balkans: Cholera Epidemic, from 'Le Petit Journal', 1st December 1912 (litho) by French School (20th century) back bl. Science & Society Picture Library: Science Museum back cra. Science Photo Library: St Mary's Hospital Medical School front clb. Still Pictures: Shehzad Noorani inside front bl. The Wellcome Institute Library, London: inside front crb.

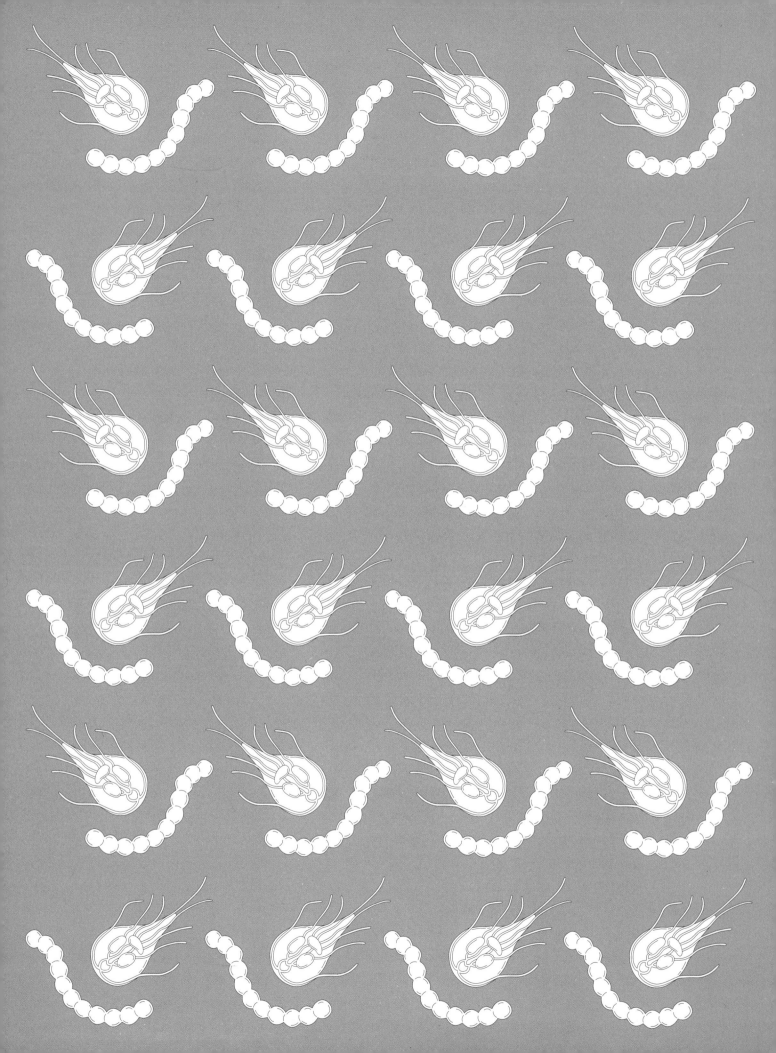